WHAT WORKS IN REDUCING INEQUALITIES IN CHILD HEALTH?

Second edition

Helen Roberts

First published in Great Britain in 2000 by Barnardo's, Tanners Lane, Barkingside, Ilford, Essex, IG6 1QG.
This edition published 2012 by The Policy Press.
© The Policy Press 2012

The Policy Press
University of Bristol
Fourth Floor
Beacon House
Queen's Road
Bristol BS8 1QU
UK
t: +44 (0)117 331 4054
f: +44 (0)117 331 4093
tpp-info@bristol.ac.uk
www.policypress.co.uk

North American office:
The Policy Press
c/o The University of Chicago Press
1427 East 60th Street
Chicago, IL 60637, USA
t: +1 773 702 7700 • f: +1 773-702-9756
sales@press.uchicago.edu • www.press.uchicago.edu

British Library Cataloguing in Publication Data
A catalogue record for this book is available from the British Library.

Library of Congress Cataloging-in-Publication Data
A catalog record for this book has been requested.

ISBN 978 1 84742 996 4 paperback
ISBN 978 1 84742 997 1 hardcover

Cover design by Qube Design Associates, Bristol
Front cover: image kindly supplied by Angela Martin
Printed and bound in Great Britain by Hobbs, Southampton
The Policy Press uses environmentally responsible print partners.

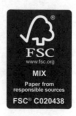

For Rodney Barker
and our children and their children

Contents

Tables and figures

Figures

Tables

Acknowledgements

Time is a scarce commodity for those of us lucky enough to be in work. Sharing that time is a gift. Colleagues who commented, provided data, or made suggestions include Lisa Arai, Audrey Brown, Ian Basnett, Ian Butler, Kalipso Chalkidou, David Collison, Katherine Curtis-Tyler, Luise Dawson, Anne Goymer, Ron Gray, Judith Harwin, Jennifer Hollowell, Jenny Kurinczuk, Catherine Law, Kristin Liabo, Patricia Lucas, Gerri McAndrew, Di McNeish, Karen Melton, Guy Palmer, Heather Payne, Douglas Simkiss, Mike Stein, Madeleine Stevens, James Thomas and Harriet Ward. I have learned a great deal from my colleagues at the National Institute for Health and Clinical Excellence (NICE), from the Canadian Institutes of Health Research-funded International Collaboration on Complex Interventions led by Penny Hawe and from the Cochrane Public Health Group led by Liz Waters. I owe them all a huge debt, particularly since I suspect I may not always have done justice to their insights.

I am grateful for permission to reproduce tables and figures whose provenance is acknowledged in the text.

Although the family is now rarely a location for the formal organisation of work, I have benefited from both the intellectual and domestic support of my husband Rodney Barker. Without Ben Barker's advisory and culinary visits, there would have been no book. He, Hannah, Polly and Tom Barker have, as ever, provided a structure and narrative to family life, and their friends, partners and children a constant source of amusement.

I was fortunate enough to spend the decade leading up to the turn of the century leading R&D in the children's charity Barnardo's, asking (among other things) what works for children? My work included a report which was the predecessor to this book. Once it became out of date, Barnardo's readily agreed to allow me to draw on it for the current work. I am grateful to those acknowledged in my original report who allowed me to draw on joint work and to my former colleagues in Barnardo's for their encouragement. I warmly acknowledge the part they play not only as a provider of services but also in pressing to have outcomes for children on the policy agenda, and as leaders of the pack in terms of the use of research evidence in child social care.

I completed the final stages of this book while a Visiting Fellow at All Souls College, Oxford. I am grateful to the Warden, Fellows, Manciple, Bursar, the Fellows' secretary Humaira Erfan-Ahmed and all the college staff to have had the opportunity to work in such unaccustomed splendour.

My publishers have been a model of encouragement. I thank them, in particular Karen Bowler, Sylvia Potter, my meticulous copy editor, and the anonymous referees. Angela Martin's cartoons, like the work of the poet Piet Hein, convey the joy of the fullness of life. I also thank Terence Stephenson for his foreword, and Russell Viner for sharing his room in University College London, which may be less splendid than All Souls, but which has a charm of its own.

Acknowledgements

Foreword

We know that social influences on health are far greater than medical ones. In 2007, a UNICEF report suggested that the well-being of children and young people in the UK was worse than that in many other economically advanced nations. However, most of the factors which the UNICEF report measured were determined to a greater extent by social factors than by medical ones. One of the most pernicious factors in society which seems to impair children's health and well-being is inequality.

Fortunately there remains a large section of society who believe in equality of opportunity. Since young children particularly cannot create their own opportunities, society and the state have to play a part in this as well as the family.

If anything, in the UK over the last decade, inequalities have got wider. We look enviously at neighbouring countries in Europe and wonder why their societies seem to function more coherently and why children and young people growing up there score better on measures of well-being.

Helen Roberts has written a fine book which examines why inequalities arise in developed societies and, more importantly, what can be done to try to reduce these and improve the health and well-being of children and young people. This debate is not so dramatic or emotive as those around open heart surgery, genetic testing of the unborn or organ donation. However, the issues which Helen Roberts raises affect far more children. I would commend this book to every reader who would like to see a better society for our children in the future.

Professor Terence Stephenson
President, Royal College of Paediatrics and Child Health

Preface

Health is not bought
With a chemist's pill
Nor saved by the surgeon's knife.
Health is not only the absence of ills
But the fight for the fullness of life.

Piet Hein (1905-96)

Health matters to children, families and communities. It also matters to policy makers and politicians. At the individual level, the plight of a sick child, at the community level, the fate of a local hospital, and at a population level, the availability or otherwise of a vaccine, attract ready media attention. Inequalities on the other hand, tend to be less attractive as headline grabbers. As a colleague put it: "Poverty is bad for your health. Well fancy that!" But the consequences of neglecting inequalities in health are as dire as those of ignoring acute health problems. Children born into poverty and disadvantage miss out on important opportunities for health gain, and accumulate health risks as they grow into adulthood.

With that in mind, the reader I have tried to imagine is the policy maker, practitioner, or student who not only wants to know something about inequalities in child health, but in a climate of budget austerity in many parts of the wealthier world, wants to know what might be done to improve health and reduce inequalities. The UK has an unrivalled reputation in terms of describing, theorising and understanding inequalities in health. Theory is important if we are to understand problems, but it is not enough.

While in the UK funding for public health research in the widest sense is strengthening the evidence base, it is likely to take some time before there is the same volume of evidence which has transformed clinical practice and survival rates for children, with five-year survival for leukaemia tripling since the 1970s. This shows that things do not have to be the way they are. There is no reason why the worse-off children should not have the same life chances as the best-off. Inequalities in health are damaging not only to the poorest children, but to us all.

Helen Roberts
London, 2012

ONE

Introduction

Investing in child public health is potentially the most important – and most effective – commitment any society can make to its future.

Inequalities in child health remain a problem even in wealthy countries such as the UK. While there has been progress in improving the health of the poorest, there is still some way to go in narrowing health gaps and reducing the health gradient. A move to an austerity climate worldwide risks not only impeding progress but undermining what has been gained.

The background of recent policy is best understood alongside an awareness of tensions between different ways of approaching problems. There is dispute, for instance, about whether universal or targeted services are the best way to address inequalities in health. Is it better to concentrate resources on the poorest, or to provide better resources for all? As Graham and Kelly (2004:10) put it '"what works" to improve the life chances and health prospects of poorer groups may not have the magnitude of effect necessary to bring them closer to the population average – or to reduce wider social and health inequalities. Being clear about what is being tackled should be integral to the development and delivery of policies to promote equity in health.' But there is no simple vaccine against poverty. Effective remedies involve addressing tax and benefits, education, employment, housing, the environment, transport and pollution. Health services are part of this picture, but by no means the major part.

At an individual and community level, social interventions are complex and like medical interventions, capable of doing harm as well as good. They need to be subject to as much evaluation as pharmaceuticals, if not more, before, during and after implementation.

Inequalities and health

We live longer than we did 50 years ago, fewer babies die at or shortly after birth, and there are fewer childhood deaths. But there remain unacceptable inequalities in health between rich and poor. Attention to inequalities in health is by no means new, but a resurgence in both science and policy offers new opportunities to act on the basis of a growing body of evidence.

Recent policy interest in inequalities in health is illustrated by a range of reports including, but not confined to, the Working Group on Inequalities in Health (1980), also known as the 'Black report', the 'Acheson report' (Acheson, 1998), the work of the Marmot Review (2010) and the Field (2010) and Allen (2011) reports. Given the most recent focus, it can be difficult to recall that until relatively recently, attention to inequalities in health was both marginal and marginalised.

It is a strength of this body of work, and the research on which it is based, that even given changes in government, the days when inequalities in health were branded 'variations' seem to be over.

There is now a very substantial body of work on theoretical, methodological and policy issues in relation to inequalities in health. What this book focuses on is an accessible overview for the non-cognoscenti, and examples of what works, or appears to work, in practice. Outlined here is the extent to which we have evidence that some interventions are more effective than others in improving health and reducing health inequalities, and the extent to which this knowledge is used, or discarded in favour of other imperatives. Having the evidence is only part of the picture. Having the political will and the combination of knowledge and skills to implement programmes or interventions which reduce inequalities is key to creating fair shares in child health. While the book has a health title, many things which have the potential to reduce health inequalities are not at first sight health-related. Support to children and their families in the early years, education and training, support for parents in and out of employment, housing and a whole range of fiscal measures may lie outside the health system, but bring well-documented health gains.

Evidence-informed practice is about ensuring that in so far as we are able given our current state of knowledge, interventions in the lives of children do as much good and as little harm as possible. The focus of this book is largely the UK, where the devolved countries and differing regions may have differing levels of problems in relation to alcohol, drugs and obesity, different levels of employment and housing, and different levels of integration of health and social care. In the case of the nations, there may be different policies on important issues, and different levels of investment in relation to reducing inequality. In recent years, infant mortality has fallen most in Wales and least in Northern Ireland, with McCormick and Harrop (2010) suggesting that devolution provides a virtual 'policy laboratory' to better understand policy and regional differences. Hirsch (2008) takes the comparative element further, setting out proposals for reducing childhood poverty in the UK to the level of the best in Europe. Notwithstanding this (largely) UK focus, much of the material here is of relevance to other middle- and high-income countries.

Described in what follows are some of the inequalities in child health which blight young lives, and examples of where there is good evidence that interventions make a difference. The collection and analysis of evidence is better in some areas than others, and we probably know a little more about the effectiveness of early interventions, for instance, than about those in middle or later childhood. Some kinds of intervention are more susceptible to robust evaluation than others, giving us more confidence in adopting them (or stopping them if they are shown to cause harm). Others may never have been evaluated at all, and it is important to bear in mind that no evidence of effect is not the same thing as evidence of no effect. The National Health Service (NHS) in the UK for instance, was not set up following a series of pilots, randomised controlled trials (RCTs) and meta-analyses. As the epidemiologist Jerry Morris put it: 'The 1940s was the generation that said "Yes we can." You need a national health service? You go out and do it' (Kuper, 2009).

The book covers health in its broadest sense – physical, mental and emotional health and well-being. It also considers the *determinants* of health – the causes of the causes of good or poor health.

Included are:

- Some of the methods which help us judge the effectiveness of an intervention. How can we know what works when faced with a barrage of conflicting studies? Should we give greater weight to some kinds of evidence than others? Are there things we routinely do in childhood with the intention of doing good which don't in fact make any difference, or which even make matters worse? What part can cost-effectiveness studies play?
- Interventions in pregnancy, early life and the pre-school period. This is an area where a relatively large amount of scientific work has been done, and where we have strong evidence of the effectiveness of some interventions.
- Interventions in childhood and adolescence.
- Interventions intended to keep children safe from accidental injury, a major childhood killer.
- Interventions with groups we know to be particularly vulnerable, in particular, children looked after by the state and disabled children.
- Interventions that tackle the causes of the causes.
- A resource list for those seeking research evidence and its links to policy, and/or those who want to contribute to the evidence agenda themselves.

It will be clear that what is covered is by no means exhaustive. This is in part because the evidence base of 'what works' remains patchy, and where the evidence itself is most solid, often draws on research from countries whose systems and child outcomes may be very different from ours (and by no means always better). Despite wide-ranging trawls, it has not always been easy to find good examples of current practice in the field based on robust research evidence. This may be in part because, as well as a 'push' to use good evidence in the provision of services, there can be a countervailing pressure, sometimes more attractive to creative and imaginative practitioners, to be innovative. Indeed, funding will sometimes depend on innovation, which can be a very strong disincentive to simply use the best of what is already known. In these cases, just as the National Institute for Health and Clinical Excellence (NICE) sometimes makes a recommendation of 'only in research' where a new technology looks promising but the evidence is insufficiently strong, there may be a 'middle way' for those developing innovative services for children to build on the best of existing evidence while working with research partners to evaluate both process and outcomes for children.

What are the causes of the causes of ill health and inequalities in health?

Germs and genetics are important factors, but so are social class, gender, ethnicity, disability, sexuality and our geographical context. Housing, employment, transport, education and the wider environment are also elements with a key influence on health and inequalities in health.

A World Health Organization poster caption asks: 'Why treat people without changing what makes them sick?',[1] and defines the social determinants of health as including the conditions in which people are born, grow, live, work and age, as well as the health system. These circumstances are shaped by the distribution of money, power and resources at global, national and local levels, which are themselves influenced by policy choices. It is the social determinants of health which are principally responsible for health inequalities – the unfair and avoidable differences in health status seen within and between countries.

What do health inequalities mean for children?

In better-off countries, we almost never see children going without shoes and most children in middle- or high-income countries do not go hungry. Few children live on the streets. But inequalities in health are a problem not just for the worst off, but for all of us. There are (at least) two ways of looking at inequalities in health and what we might do about them. One is to concentrate on the gap between the best off and the worst off. The other is to think about the slope between those at the bottom of the pile and those at the top – 'the gradient' – since differences will usually be seen all the way up. Perhaps one of the clearest examples of this relates to a long-term study of British civil servants (Marmot et al., 1991), which showed not only those in the lowest grade such as messengers having much higher mortality than those at the top of the civil service, but also that there were differences all the way up the finely graded civil service hierarchy. Even those at the very pinnacle do not entirely benefit from their situation, given that for many, whatever their political views, it is deeply disturbing to live in a society where there is an unfair distribution of health and well-being.

Inequalities in health do not just relate to socioeconomic status, though since this is where we tend to have the most consistent data, it is the dimension most frequently referred to in this book. Other dimensions of inequality can relate to whole countries. Figure 7.2. for example, shows differences in child well-being in countries which are more and less equal. Ethnicity is a further dimension, and Figure 3.2, for instance, shows inequalities in infant mortality by ethnic group. Children looked after by the state and children brought up in private households also have different life chances, resulting in inequalities in health and life more broadly.

---

[1] www.who.int/social_determinants/en/

4

In addressing inequalities in health, we can put efforts into improving the health of the poorest, trying to close the gap between those at the top and those at the bottom, or we can try to alter the slope or the gradient so that people all the way up are doing better (although there will still be a gap between the best and the worst off). Graham and Kelly (2004:10) suggest that each of these adds a further layer to the policy challenge. As they point out, improving the health of the poorest is a goal in line with policy trends, whereas narrowing the gap and reducing the health gradient are more challenging.

Inequalities in health are closely tied to wealth (and poverty). Children born into poverty are more likely than their better-off neighbours to:

- die in the first year of life
- be born small, be born early, or both
- be bottle fed
- die or be seriously injured in a childhood accident
- smoke and have a parent who smokes
- become overweight or obese
- have or father children before they are ready to
- parent alone
- die younger.

But these outcomes are not just true of the poorest children – mortality, breastfeeding and accidental death in childhood and other health-related factors all form a gradient from the poorest doing worst to the least poor tending to do best.

While these are clearly matters of concern, children and young people are not simply 'objects of concern'. They are active citizens with views and rights. Each chapter makes reference to the views of children and young people, and draws on studies where their voices are heard. As Mayall (1995) suggests, it is critical to understand children's own experiences in evaluating services. While abstract issues such as inequalities in health are not, on the whole, ones which children would themselves raise using those terms, they have an early understanding of injustice, as anyone familiar with the phrase "That's not fair!" will know. Even at an early age, they can be aware of the links between health, wealth and well-being. A study carried out by Newman (2000) asked a large sample of junior school children, 'if you had one wish come true, what would it be?' Responses showed both generosity and altruism:

> 'If I had a wish I would wish that my house was not being repossessed.'
> (Girl, 10)

> 'I wish I would not suffer from asthma so my mother doesn't have to do so much dusting. I wish my dad could have more time off work.'
> (Boy, 10)

'That my family could be safe all their lives in a safe street.' (Boy, 11)

'I wish that I could help the poor people who haven't got no food water or nothing' (Girl, 8)

'A big house for all the homeless and money for the homeless and some clothes and shoes because it is nasty for people to be on streets.' (Girl, 11)

Why do inequalities matter?

Poverty and inequality in early childhood cast a long shadow forward, and many of the problems which they cause are cumulative. This means that although death in childhood is now rare, the consequences of having a poor start in life are more insidious. Meantime, problems in the here and now include children already disadvantaged through disability or chronic illness being doubly disadvantaged because of extra strains on the family income, and time spent accessing and attending services.

Despite medical and social welfare advances, inequalities in childhood remain stark. But while measures of the health effects of poverty have been used to some effect in influencing policy (Marmot et al., 2010; Whitehead and Popay, 2010), metrics tend to have more traction when drawing attention to calls for extra incubators, extra surgeons, or extra high-dependency beds. Just as important as the numbers game in constructing a narrative to support investment in reducing inequalities in health is a seam of qualitative work describing the texture of the lives of mothers and children living in poverty (Graham, 1993a; Bostock, 1998; Dearlove, 1999). Children's own experiences of poverty tend to be less fully described, in part because the poorest parents try to shield their children from its worst effects (Middleton et al., 1997), a finding confirmed in a study of a child's eye view of social difference a decade later (Sutton et al., 2007).

Poverty, inequality and the NHS

The link between early events and later outcomes – and the recognition that interventions at crucial points may affect this – has long been understood. The Book of Daniel describes an experiment in which children were given pulses to eat and water to drink, rather than the king's wine and meat. While present day nutritionists might be astonished by the speed of the effect, good nutrition was clearly established as a helpful intervention by finding that after only 10 days, the countenances of the experimental group 'were fairer and fatter in flesh than all the children which did eat the portion of the King's meat' (Holy Bible).

In the early 1940s, following the publication of *Birth, poverty and wealth* (Titmuss, 1943), newspapers reported 'Poor folks' babies stand less chance', and 'Babies beware of poor parents'. Titmuss had suggested that children's deaths were related to the occupations of their fathers, and that the gap between the life chances of working-class and middle-class infants was increasing. Some found his conclusions unpalatable. A reviewer for the *Evening Citizen* suggested that the book ignored 'the criminal ignorance and neglect of many mothers', inclined to give their babies 'fish and chips, pickles, strong tea, lollipops, chocolate biscuits and toffee apples' (Oakley, 1996:190). A review of the BMA's Growing up in Britain asked the same question, but also suggested a plausible answer. 'Why do children from poor families consume such a lot of sweets, fizzy drinks, milk and white bread? Penny for penny, a chocolate bar provides more calories than carrots, even from a market stall' (Thurlbeck, 2000:809).

Over half a century after Titmuss's publication, press coverage of work on poverty and inequality could still be sceptical. When the children's charity Barnardo's published Richard Wilkinson's *Unfair shares* (Wilkinson, 1994) the *Guardian* (1994) urged that it should inform policy, while the editor of the *British Medical Journal* highlighted a *Daily Mail* article which concluded: 'Rich or poor, life is getting better ... the vast majority are doing well and don't need welfare' (Smith, 1996). While some of this rhetoric continues, there is a more broadly based political acceptance of inequalities as a problem which needs to be addressed. Before becoming Prime Minister, David Cameron, in his Hugo Young memorial lecture in 2009 said:

> The size, scope and role of the state is of course the scene of a vigorous political debate. But ... it is pointless to draw dividing lines where none exist. Ask anyone of any political colour the kind of country they want to see and they'll say a Britain that is richer, that is safer, that is greener but perhaps most important to us all, a country that is fairer and where opportunity is more equal.
>
> ... the incredible wealth of the City exists side-by-side with some of the poorest neighbourhoods in our country. For every tube station along the Jubilee Line, from Westminster to the East End, Londoners living in those areas lose almost an entire year of expected life. Bringing these two worlds closer is a multi-faceted endeavour: moral, social, and of course economic.
>
> Research by Richard Wilkinson and Katie Pickett has shown that among the richest countries, it's the more unequal ones that do worse according to almost every quality of life indicator. In *The spirit level*, they show that per capita GDP is much less significant for a country's life expectancy, crime levels, literacy and health than the size of the gap between the richest and poorest in the population. So the best indicator of a country's rank on these measures of general well-being is not the difference in wealth between them, but the difference in wealth within them. (Cameron, 2009)

A change of rhetoric does not of course, necessarily presage a change of policy, and it may well be argued that engagement in scientific debates slows rather than hastens policy development and political action. In addition, as Mackenbach (2011) points out, health inequalities can only be reduced substantially if governments have a democratic mandate to make the necessary policy changes, if demonstrably effective policies can be developed, and if these policies are implemented on the scale needed to reach the overall targets.

One thing which has not changed is that now as in the 1940s, mothers – still the major carers for children – continue to attract adverse press and sometimes professional comment, with suggestions that the main need for change lies with them. Their children can be portrayed as suffering when they go out to work and when they do not. Their diets are not sensible, their discipline lacking, their parenting skills wanting. The 2011 riots in London saw two kinds of mother narrative, the bad mother, usually single and indifferent to her children running riot and the feisty mother marching her miscreant child to the police station. Such portrayals come in spite of evidence that the majority of mothers living in poverty protect and promote the health of their children under the most unpromising conditions (Roberts et al., 1995; Kempson, 1996). The harm done by failing to affirm the achievements of the majority of good mothers, and to recognise the barriers and obstacles to good mothering, sometimes invisible to professionals, cannot be underestimated.

When considering health and ill health in the UK, the NHS is often considered the principal contributor. We like to think of ourselves as one of the more privileged nations in which to bring up children. We have a health service of which most Britons are justly proud, and the UK is a country where health outcomes for children are rather better than those in countries to which we sometimes look for policy ideas and research evidence. Medical care is free at the point of use, and there are no prescription charges for under 16s. There has been some change for the better since Tudor Hart (1971), a GP in Wales, described in the *Lancet* the inverse care law, whereby medical care was lowest where the needs of the population were highest. A decade and a half later, Tudor Hart (1988) could write: 'it is better, much better than it was, but still far below what it should be'.

As the Department of Health's strategy for public health in England points out (Department of Health, 2010), health care services probably account for only about a third of the improvements to life expectancy (Bunker, 2001), the remainder of the improvements lying in 'changing people's lifestyles and removing health inequalities'. However, in one crucial respect, the NHS plays a key part. Universal access to health care, free at the point of delivery, is an important intervention (Arblaster et al., 1996:101). So while it would be mistaken to see the NHS as the key player in addressing inequalities, there is a large body of evidence on the ways in which the NHS, alongside advances in housing and education, has improved the health of the nation.

Death and disease in childhood

Death in childhood in the UK is now uncommon. A decade or so into the twenty-first century in the UK, infectious diseases have all but disappeared as causes of childhood death. A child dying from measles or pneumonia is a rarity. This is in part as a result of successful immunisation against common childhood diseases which were killers in the past. An example is given in the next box of an initiative in Tower Hamlets to raise their immunisation rates.

Improving the coverage of the childhood immunisation programme in Tower Hamlets

The reported rates of all vaccination uptake in London have consistently been below the England averages and there have been concerns in the capital about an outbreak of measles. Achieving herd immunity across the childhood immunisation programme has been a long-term priority of NHS Tower Hamlets.

Research commissioned by the public health directorate identified that one of the key barriers to parents attending vaccination appointments was the lack of reminders to inform them when the vaccinations were due. A 'whole systems' approach was required to improve the coverage levels of vaccinations in the 0–5 years programme. Obtaining robust data from primary care was a crucial element. Following this, a number of interventions were put in place, including:

- capitalising on the network structure (clusters of 4/5 practices), a primary care commissioning investment, to deliver this service;
- developing a comprehensive call and recall system at a network level;
- a list cleaning exercise;
- adoption of a local enhanced service to incentivise obtaining 95% levels of uptake;
- training and supporting network teams to implement the immunisation programme;
- targeting individual networks and practices to identify initiatives to make improvements to the uptake.

Published results from NHS London for the end of the fourth quarter of 2010/11 show Tower Hamlets to have achieved the highest coverage level of the childhood vaccination schedule across the capital. The most recent data indicate that for the first year set of vaccinations, coverage has increased from 91% (2009/10) to 97%.

Luise Dawson, personal communication, July 2011 (see also Cockman et al., 2011)

In terms of child deaths, although numbers have fallen overall, accidental death remains a major childhood killer, with a steep social class gradient illustrating that it is not the random events that the term 'accident' may imply, but a matter of who you are born to, and where you are born. Child deaths in house fires have the steepest social class gradient of all (Edwards et al., 2006).

Figure 1.1 shows the steep decline in childhood deaths, but also that the decline has been much less steep in adolescence and early adulthood, where injury from accidents and suicide remain an important risk.

Figure 1.1: Age-specific mortality in England and Wales: 1960–2000

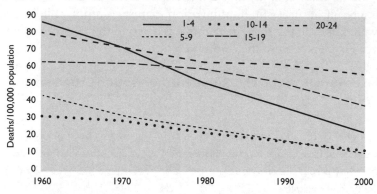

Reprinted with permission from BMJ Publishing Group; from Viner, R. M. and Barker, M. 'Young people's health: the need for action', *British Medical Journal*, 14 April 2005, 330: 901 doi: 10.1136/bmj.330.7496.901.

In terms of disability, Spencer et al. (2010) report that the poorest children are 3.5 times more likely to have a limiting longstanding illness or disability than the best off. They point out that if all children and young people were to have the same rate of longstanding illness and disability as the most advantaged group, there would be a 41% decrease across the population.

The most comprehensive picture we have of children's health still comes from the Department of Health surveys conducted in 1995–97 (Prescott-Clarke and Primatesta, 1998). At that time, just over a quarter of boys and just under a quarter of girls aged 2–15 years reported a longstanding illness, with 10% indicating that it limited their activities in some way. Parents spoke for children aged 2–12; 13-year-olds and above spoke for themselves. Descriptions of general health, however, were much more positive, with 90% of parents of 2- to 15-year-olds describing their general health as 'good' or 'very good'. In 2000, 81% of children were reported by their parent or guardian to be in good health; 15% as having fairly good health; and 3% as not having good health (Rickards et al., 2004).

In terms of mental health, the Office for National Statistics reports that in 2004, 1 in 10 children and young people aged 5–16 had a clinically recognisable mental health problem. Children with mental health problems, particularly those with emotional and conduct disorders, are much more likely than other children to have time off school. The prevalence of mental health problems was greater among children living in low-income high-unemployment areas (15%) compared with affluent areas (7%) (Green et al., 2005).

Policy reports and the importance of prevention

Influential in putting health inequalities on to the agenda was the Black report (Working Group on Inequalities in Health, 1980), and in keeping it there, an inquiry chaired by Sir Donald Acheson, a former chief medical officer, resulting in the publication of the *Independent inquiry into inequalities in health* (Acheson, 1998). The story of the Black report coming to prominence is one which nicely illustrates the law of unintended consequences. In a clumsy attempt to muffle the findings of a committee appointed by a Labour Secretary of State in 1977, the incoming government scheduled publication for the August Bank Holiday in 1980, with a print run of only 260 copies. The attempted sidelining ensured far wider publicity than it might otherwise have had. In a splendid example of what happens when you fail to learn from history, in 1987, when a follow-up report, *The health divide* was published (HEC, 1987) it had its official press launch at the Health Education Council cancelled. The launch was reconvened round the corner below a music shop in Soho, London. Once again, it caught press attention in a way which it might not otherwise have done.

It was the Black and then the Acheson reports which set the scene for the following decades, and sufficient time has passed to have a sense of the extent to which some of their recommendations have been mainstreamed. The most important thing that those of us with an interest in reducing inequalities in child health can take from the Acheson report is that the areas identified for action were not 'medical' ones. Despite the fact that the inquiry was chaired by one of the country's most senior doctors, reporting to the Secretary of State for Health, most of what was covered by the recommendations were not tasks for the NHS. The report concentrated on diagnosis and general policy treatment rather than detailed practice prescriptions. It pulled together some of the most robust research, and made three major policy recommendations:

- Policies likely to affect health should be evaluated in terms of their impact on health inequalities.
- A high priority should be given to the health of families with children.
- Steps should be taken to reduce income inequalities and improve the living standards of poor households.

Of the recommendations in the report, 10 were of particular relevance in reducing health inequalities for children and young people, and notwithstanding the reports which have come since, are worth rehearsing here, since, although there is some way to go, there has been quite substantial progress, particularly in terms of early childhood policy. These are:

- reduction in poverty in women of childbearing age, expectant mothers, young children and older people by increasing benefits in cash or kind;

- the development of high-quality pre-school education so that it meets, in particular, the needs of disadvantaged families;
- measures to encourage walking and cycling and the separation of pedestrians and cyclists from motor vehicles;
- policies which reduce poverty in families with children by promoting material support, removing barriers to work for parents who wish to combine work with parenting, and enabling those who want to be full-time parents to do so;
- an integrated policy for the provision of affordable, high-quality day care and pre-school education with extra resources for disadvantaged communities;
- policies which improve the health and nutrition of women of childbearing age and their children, prioritising the elimination of food poverty and the prevention and reduction of obesity;
- policies which increase breastfeeding;
- policies which promote social and emotional support for parents and children;
- consideration of minority ethnic groups in needs assessment, resource allocation and health care planning and provision;
- policies which reduce psychosocial ill health in young women in disadvantaged circumstances, particularly those caring for young children.

Some of the policy reports which followed are referred to in the final chapter and the Appendix, but it was Black and Acheson which began to move inequalities in health from the margins to the mainstream.

What works?

What Works? as a title should perhaps come with its own health warning. While it is possible to give strong guidance in some areas on what works in child public health and social care, it would be arrogant to do more than describe what works, or is likely to work, in a particular context at a particular time. While there is growing evidence of the kinds of intervention likely to be effective, our knowledge of what is working well on the ground needs to be strengthened. Evidence-informed policy and practice is about ensuring that the interventions made in the lives of children do as much good (and as little harm) as possible, given our current state of knowledge.

The history of intervening in children's lives has been mixed. While no one can doubt the value of many of the efforts of those who founded the children's charities, or set about ensuring universal education, by no means every effort intended to improve children's lives has been unambiguously beneficial. The development of a robust knowledge base to underpin effective services and an understanding of how that knowledge gets used in practice is not just a professional issue, it is also a rights issue. Children and families have a right to expect that those providing services will operate on the basis of the best of what is already known. This includes not just conventional research knowledge, but also knowledge gained from children and families who use the available services.

What is an intervention?

'Interventions' in this context are actions undertaken with the intention of bringing about a benefit. It is easier to view inserting grommets into a child's ears, a course of antibiotics or a tonsillectomy as health interventions; more difficult is a parenting support programme, school milk, school meals or free bus travel for children. It is probably easier to find evidence-informed practice guidance on amputation or appendectomy than it is to find the same kinds of information on accident prevention, acting on obesity, or adoption, in part because building the evidence base in child public health and social care is possibly more complex, and certainly less well-funded, than clinical research.

The interventions which are the most broadly effective in reducing inequalities in health and in life include tax and benefits systems, employment policies and practices, including of course the employment and conditions of those working with children, and resource allocation within and between the services which impact on children and families.

Individualised interventions such as parent education, home visiting and mentoring, as at least some of their proponents and evaluators would be the first to agree, tend to be black boxes with a great many unanswered questions about what specific type of intervention, if any, may be effective and, if so, how and under what conditions. Some interventions, powerfully described by their proponents, can gain momentum because they have strong face validity. They look like the sort of things that should work, our 'gut' feelings tell us that they will work and we want them to work. Not only may this result in premature roll-out on the basis of insufficient evidence, but it may be difficult to stop or change direction once programmes have been launched. For that and other reasons, it is important to focus on the dynamic properties of the context into which the intervention is introduced and the part played by practitioners and relationship building (Hawe et al., 2009; Riley and Hawe, 2009).

What makes for a successful intervention?

The most successful interventions in reducing inequalities in health are likely to be those at a national or even supra-national level, but many decisions about resources and interventions are made regionally or locally.

The next box gives a checklist of more pragmatic questions to be considered when designing an intervention, and the kinds of evidence which it might be reasonable for users to expect:

The intervention
- Has an assessment of needs been done to help shape the intervention?
- Is the intended intervention acceptable, and culturally and educationally appropriate?
- Have people on the receiving end been involved in the design and development of the intervention?
- Will the intervention be delivered in the same way to everyone or flexibly delivered?

Setting and participants
- Is the setting accessible to, and accepted by those receiving it?
- Would it be more appropriate to deliver the intervention to individuals or to groups? If to groups, what might be their best composition and size?

Delivering the intervention
- Who might be the most appropriate agent to deliver the intervention, for example, health professional, teacher, community volunteer, trained peer?
- How readily do those receiving the intervention identify with those delivering it, and what personal skills, training and support might they need?

Support materials/resources
- If the intervention requires the use of written or audiovisual materials, what are the most appropriate materials given the language abilities, literacy skills and preferences of those receiving it?
- Would the provision of assistance with transport and/or childcare make it easier for people to attend the health care intervention?

Adapted from Arblaster et al. (1996:100)

Universal and targeted interventions

Given the unequal distribution of ill health among children, it may appear to make sense to target interventions at those in greatest need. But there are also good public health arguments for universal services. 'Targeting' and 'homing in on risk factors' use the militaristic language of problem solving, but the success of doing things this way depends on our being very clear on just who the target population is, and then working out which interventions will be effective. This is true whether the problem is road traffic injuries, respiratory disease or children and young people using illegal substances.

'Targeting' is comforting to those of us who might occasionally eat too much, drink too much or fail to exercise, because it *isn't aimed at us*. Our habits and activities are normal. It's those at the extreme who need attention. What is more, targeting isn't just a comfort to the slightly over-indulgent. It may also provide some (possibly temporary) comfort to the Treasury and less lofty purchasers of services intended to divert unhealthy, antisocial or simply misguided behaviours by clever risk assessment and precise focusing. Theoretically, targeting will be cheaper than measures aimed at whole populations. But only if it works. Targeting may seem cheaper and more efficient than universal provision, but this is only the case if assumptions about its effectiveness, and our ability to target the right people, are correct. If targeting carries a stigma, then it may be at best ineffective, as some of the eligible children and parents will avoid the service, or at worst harmful, as children who used to have to queue separately for free school meals can testify.

The attraction of a universal approach to a child public health issue can be illustrated with a medical analogy. Writing in the *British Medical Journal* on high blood pressure, alcohol use and obesity, Geoffrey Rose and Simon Day (1990) pointed out that traditional prevention strategies aim to eliminate the high 'tail' of the distribution, but not to interfere with the rest of the population. Rose and Day found in samples representing 52 populations in 32 countries that average blood pressure predicted the number of hypertensive people; the average weight predicted the number of obese people and the average alcohol intake the number of heavy drinkers. Obesity may be considered a bad thing, but average weight, until very recently, was considered acceptable, even in overweight populations. In practice, dealing with a problem by dealing with the tail alone is likely to be ineffective. The statistical 'tail', they point out, is part of the animal. The way most people eat, drink and behave, even if harmless to themselves, may affect how others, more vulnerable, may act.

A number of studies of child weight suggest that parents from 'big' families tend to normalise size (Baughcum et al., 1998; Reifsnider et al (2000) in Lucas et al., 2007):

'you look at me and his father, so he's not gonna be little either'

'he's finally taking the form he's supposed to have'

As we become more overweight as a society, bigger children may seem more normal, despite the evidence that overweight and obesity are bad for their long-term health and general well-being. Figures 1.2 and 1.3 illustrate the way in which shifting the mean may be preferable as a method, because it is non-stigmatising, it affects a greater number and it changes the way in which problems are viewed.

Research, policy and practice

Research can help us understand the social world; understand at least in part, why positive and negative events occur in the lives of some and not others; and understand the effects and relative effectiveness of interventions on these events. However, research is only one source of knowledge, and in terms of the policies and practices of organisations intervening in the lives of vulnerable people, not necessarily the most influential. It has to compete with other sources (some more reliable than others) such as personal experience, the influence of colleagues, the media, organisational policies and procedures, custom and practice (Barnardo's R&D Team, 2000).

Most requests for service funding – setting up a new service, or retaining funds for a more established one – will come with some kind of evidence that the service is worthwhile. Sometimes the evidence is strong, sometimes less so. It is

Figure 1.2: Targeted intervention

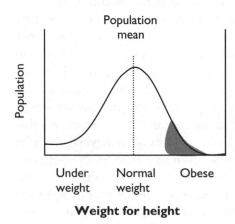

Figure 1.3: Shifting the mean

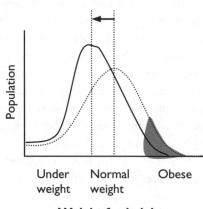

frequently difficult for those commissioning services to have a clear idea of the strength of the evidence in a particular field. How can we ensure that mediocre or poor research, persuasively presented, does not create 'noise' which drowns out more robust research whose results may be more equivocal?

The Appendix provides links to some of the more reliable evidence sources, including NHS Evidence, which deals with both health and social care, the Cochrane Collaboration, which is concerned with the preparation and maintenance of systematic reviews of health care interventions, and the Campbell Collaboration, which provides systematic reviews for sound interventions in education, social welfare and criminal justice. The Social Care Institute for Excellence (SCIE) and The Centre for Excellence and Outcomes in Children and Young People's Services (C4EO) also provide useful information, data and links.

And when there is no evidence?

While the time that it will take to establish a more complete evidence base is a short one in the history of science, it is a long time in the life of a child. Those who provide services will often give to those funding them some kind of evidence that the proposed service is an important one, and will improve matters for the population at risk. The problem is that as well as a good deal of sound research supporting or otherwise particular interventions, there is some very poor research, and some that makes claims greater than can be justified.

Interventions which we carry out without good evidence that they will be effective are, in effect, uncontrolled experiments with people's lives, though we may be loath to see it that way. The impulse to want to 'do something' is strong. But while the default position should be to build services on good evidence of what works, there will also be situations where new challenges are faced, and rapid action needed. When unaccompanied refugee children arrive from a newly conflict-ridden zone for instance, there may be little we can draw on that bears directly on their particular situation. There may though, be 'near' evidence – for instance evaluations of child refugees from other cultures, and studies of refugees and resilience. We do not, in the UK, have a good record of learning from work on the strengths of refugees, or the problems created by the thin dispersal of refugee groups (Edholm et al., 1983).

The ethical position remains to deliver services on the basis of the best of current knowledge; to acknowledge that innovation will sometimes be another word for experimentation, to keep an open mind, and to ensure that services for which evidence of effectiveness is thin are well evaluated. Simply knowing that poverty and inequality are bad for health does not get us very far. Poor people have always known that poverty is bad for you. Better-off people have always known that having sufficient money to eat well, buy decent housing and live in unpolluted areas is a good thing. For that reason, it is important not just to describe and theorise inequalities in health, but to carry out robust evaluations of interventions, and then work out how best to introduce and implement those interventions that make a positive difference.

There has long been a belief that early years work is worthwhile. Now there is sound research to show that this is so. Early years initiatives can improve health and well-being and close the health gap. Moreover, so long as they are well designed and well delivered, they provide fun in the here and now for children and parents, as well as promoting change later. Reducing inequalities need not be a bitter pill.

Key messages

- For us to make a meaningful difference to inequalities in health, we need to tackle not just health problems but the determinants of those problems – the causes of the causes. There is compelling evidence linking health and wealth.
- The health service on its own cannot tackle inequalities in child health.
- Some measures taken to improve health may widen inequalities.
- While many interventions intended to improve matters for the poorest sections of the community are targeted, there is a strong public health argument for universal services. Most poor children do not live in poor communities.
- There is not an effective intervention for every problem. This makes it important to act on the basis of those interventions with good evidence of effectiveness, and where there is no good evidence, to recognise that we are experimenting.

- Where we are experimenting, we need to evaluate well so that we can know whether we are doing good, doing harm, or using resources which will leave matters much as they were.
- 'Strong' evaluation (rather than evaluation as justification) needs to be a routine part of ethical practice.
- In our search for ways of narrowing inequalities in child health, we have things that we can learn from children and young people, who have a unique perspective on what it is to be a child.

TWO

What kinds of studies help us understand what works?

Is water fluoridation effective in reducing dental caries in children? Do children learn better in small classes? Can young offenders be 'scared straight' through tough penal measures? Can the steep social class gradient in fire-related child deaths be reduced by installing smoke alarms? What do children do when the smoke alarm goes off? What can we learn from young people who don't smoke or drink? These and other questions each require different kinds of methods to provide an answer.

While service providers may prefer to turn to the substantive chapters, students may find it helpful to engage with this one, which is directed towards readers who want to know something of the research background to making judgements about what works. The careful practitioner, manager or policy maker needs evidence (and the capacity to judge the evidence of others) in order to inform their policies or interventions. 'Research shows …' is not enough. We need to know whether the information on which policies or interventions are founded is based on good, mediocre or poor research, and what it *means*. The 'what works' agenda is about using the best available evidence from a range of methods and a range of experts, including lay experts – children and families who are on the receiving end of services. Good research, both qualitative and quantitative, allows us to have some confidence in relating a particular course of events to a particular outcome, that is, in understanding what works, might work, or seems promising.

Societies in which everything is questioned although more awkward, have benefits in terms of transparency and democratic decision making: 'An evaluative culture is an aspect of the open society. It is one in which propositions can be divided between those that are supported by evidence, and those which are not. The way to distinguish between these two types of propositions is to ask, "what is the evidence?"' (Gray, 2000:8).

There used to be a touching belief that some kinds of interventions were exempt from the sort of scrutiny that we might normally expect to be a prerequisite for messing around with other people's lives (Skrabanek, 1990). Even once it was accepted that physicians and surgeons might inadvertently do more harm than good, some areas of public health occupied a privileged place. A few leaflets, classes showing parents how to do their jobs better, giving free bus passes to children or handing out free smoke alarms: what could be the harm in that? All are interventions, but the evidence on the good they do in relation to costs, and how they might best be implemented if worthwhile is only now starting to accrue.

Not everything we might do with the intention of benefiting children is susceptible to hard-nosed research evidence of course. Many important interventions, actions and policies are matters for social value judgements, which may be informed by science, but which are not themselves the result of a scientific investigation. Jim Loach's film *Oranges and Sunshine* for instance, portrays the children who, until well into the second half of the twentieth century, were being sent overseas for a fresh start in life. Knowing what we know now about the experiences of many of these children, would we do the same thing? Surely not, despite not knowing what life would have been like for them had they not been sent overseas.

Would disabled children now be incarcerated in hospitals or other institutions, simply because they had a physical or learning disability? Probably not, since it is as difficult to see the rationale for this as it is to understand why, in the southern states of the US, it took so long for Black and White students to be educated at the same university. Simply questioning what we do, should lead us to consider harms as well as benefits from innovations which may have a strong face validity ('it sounds like a good idea').

This is not simply a matter of 'we know better now'. Current methods frequently judged adequate in evaluating interventions in children's lives might not have been much help in judging, for instance, childhood emigration policies. A social marketing approach would undoubtedly have identified a plausible narrative and considerable enthusiasm both among those responsible for sending the children overseas, those receiving them, and indeed, from some of the evidence we have, from the children themselves when offered a trip to a new country when most had never travelled beyond their own city. Had the UK's policy of sending children to New Zealand, Canada or Australia been subjected to a process evaluation, the report may well have said that the children looked well cared for, and the food, transport and child to adult ratios were adequate. But if other questions had been asked, of other people, and at other moments in the implementation of the policy, different conclusions might have been reached. Early in the history of child migration, in an early example of listening to children, one inspector got another side of the story, often missing from current policy evaluations where the question 'what goes wrong?' is left unreported. At sea, one child told him, 'We sicked all over each other.' The meaning of adoption was explained: ' 'Doption sir, is when folks get a girl to work without wages' (Doyle, 1875).

This chapter looks at how we might increase our confidence that practices and policies will do good rather than harm, and that the investments in children will improve their well-being and life chances now and in the future. The kinds of methods used to populate the evidence base have sometimes been the subject of controversy, though it is now widely agreed that there is no simple hierarchy of evidence, although ideally, new interventions will be based on systematic reviews synthesising data from different sources. Hardly surprisingly, some methods are likely to be more useful than others in answering certain types of question (Petticrew and Roberts, 2003; Glasziou et al., 2004; Rawlins, 2008). For some questions, a qualitative study will be the most useful, for some a cost–benefit study, and for some a randomised controlled trial (RCT) or cohort study. For the whole picture, more than one method is needed, which is why research synthesis is so important. Table 2.1 sets out the kinds of questions for which a particular research design might be helpful.

Interventions of the type discussed in this book tend to be not just complicated, but complex. As Shiell et al. (2008) point out, complexity has two meanings. In the first, it is a property of the intervention, and in the second a property of the system in which the intervention is implemented; this has important implications for evaluation, and in particular economic evaluation.

This means that the evidence for effectiveness has to find a way of encompassing that complexity. Referring to this problem, Rychetnik et al. (2002) ask whether and to what extent evaluative research on public health interventions can be appraised by applying well-established criteria for judging the quality of evidence in clinical practice. As they indicate, the evaluation has to distinguish between the *fidelity of the process* in assessing the success or failure of an intervention – are those intervening doing what they are supposed to? – and the *success or failure of the intervention itself*. As they point out, if an intervention is unsuccessful, evidence from the evaluation should help to determine whether it was inherently faulty (that is, failure of intervention concept or theory), or just badly delivered (failure of implementation).

The Medical Research Council (MRC) complex interventions guidelines (Craig et al., 2008; MRC, 2008) make clear that developing and evaluating complex interventions is not always a linear process and experimental designs are not always possible or practical. They warn that understanding processes, while important cannot trump understanding outcomes, but concede that complex interventions may work best if tailored to local circumstances. They suggest that reports of studies include a detailed description of the intervention to enable replication, evidence synthesis and wider implementation.

The challenge of evaluation at a local level

A number of problems face the health or social care worker or teacher who wants to assess the effectiveness of what they or their team are doing, whether this is everyday practice or a particular intervention. While the cautionary example described in the next box was first set out well over a decade ago, the approach is still frequently used in making a case, although the reader may want to consider how reliable it is.

Table 2.1: Horses for courses: different kinds of research evidence for different kinds of question

Research question	Qualitative research	Survey	Case control studies	Cohort Studies	RCTs	Quasi-experimental studies	Non-experimental evaluations	Systematic reviews
Effectiveness *Does this work? Does doing this work better than doing that?*				+	++	+		+++
Effectiveness of service delivery How does it work?	++	+					+	+++
Salience Does it matter?	++	++						+++
Safety Will it do more good than harm?	+		+	+	++	+	+	+++
Acceptability Will children/parents be willing to or want to take up the service offered?	++	+			+	+	+	+++
Cost-effectiveness Is it worth buying this service?					++			+++
Appropriateness Is this the right service for these children?	++	++						++
Quality How good is the service ?	++	++	+	+				+

Source: Petticrew and Roberts (2003 [adapted from Gray,1997])
Reprinted with permission from BMJ Publishing Group; from Petticrew, M. and Roberts, H. 'Evidence, hierarchies and typologies: horses for courses' *Journal of Epidemiology and Community Health,* 2003, 57, pp 527–9

Suppose a team wants to evaluate a discussion group aimed at improving the parenting skills of a group of parents living in poverty. The programme runs for eight weekly sessions and is considered by both the workers and parents to have been a success, at least for those who did not drop out or fail to turn up for even the first session. Their judgement is based on self-reports of the parents, the workers' observations of parents' increasing self-esteem, and improvements in the apparent well-being of the children (who have been cared for in a playgroup during the parents' discussions). Before asserting that 'groups like this work' we need to be as certain as possible that:

- improvements *have* taken place; and
- they have been brought about as a result of the discussion group.

It is difficult to do this if we do not have mechanisms for ruling out competing explanations, such as:

- The parents might have improved simply with the passage of time and increased confidence in their parenting ability. There is evidence from other fields that many problems improve spontaneously over time in two thirds of cases (see Rachman and Wilson, 1980).
  This provides a reason for considering a no-treatment control, particularly if there is a waiting list and no immediate danger, so that we can compare the effects of an intervention with a 'wait and see' approach.
- The children might have become more manageable through spending time with skilled playgroup workers.
- Other external factors might be responsible for changes, such as improved income support, additional help from social services or more help from the wider family.
- The perceived improvement in the parents might be due to their having learned the 'right' things to say in the course of the intervention, having been asked the same kind of questions at the beginning and end of the programme, and become familiar with the expectations of the workers.
- The parents who stayed might have been highly motivated and would have improved anyway. Alternatively, those parents who dropped out might have done just as well as those in the programme. We simply don't know.

Macdonald and Roberts (1995)

These would be reasonable responses to claims that a particular programme is responsible for change. They demonstrate the difficulties that arise whenever we do something that we claim produces clear outcomes, whether good or bad.

Does it work? How can we design and deliver effective services?

Many research stories of the type reported on the morning radio news have an underlying agenda. Advocates of mentoring schemes will call for more investment in mentoring; those who provide counselling services will call for more counselling; those who espouse parent education for more of that. These calls may well be justified, but how can we judge, and which are the ones which, with limited resources, will make the most meaningful differences to reducing inequalities in child health?

Evidence-informed policy and practice would suggest that we select an intervention because a review of the evidence indicates that this course of action is more likely than the alternative(s) (including doing nothing) to result in the best possible outcome for the child and/or family.

In order to answer the 'does it work?' question, some kinds of evidence are likely to be more helpful than others. Evidence-informed child public health can be seen as the process of systematically locating, critically reviewing and using research findings as the basis for interventions. As well as considering the effectiveness of interventions, evidence-informed practice is also concerned with the accuracy of diagnostic tools and strategies needed to deploy finite resources where they are most needed. How big is the problem? Is the workforce skilled up to deal with it? The answers to these questions have particular relevance when there is doubt about the best course of action in the management of a problem. Reducing inequalities in child health is such a field.

Four basic steps in identifying good evidence to underpin practice from Rosenberg and Donald (1995) are adapted here:

- Formulate questions from the perspective of end-point users. What are the issues which are making the biggest difference to children's lives according to them and to parents, teachers and others who spend a lot of time with them?
- Search the literature for relevant studies. It is still frequently the case that interventions will be built on a brief narrative review of the literature, drawing on studies which support a particular intervention, and ignoring others.
- Critically appraise the evidence for validity and usefulness. How good is the evidence, and how transferable into practice?
- Implement the findings in practice.

The final step is probably the most difficult one, and a step which is often poorly understood and frequently under-resourced. The barriers and obstacles to implementing interventions on the basis of good evidence frequently outweigh the mechanisms for doing so. The barriers to *stopping* doing something even when there is good evidence that it is not worthwhile, or may even be doing harm, may be even harder to surmount.

Systematic reviews

Anyone faced with making a decision about the effectiveness of an intervention, whether a social intervention, such as the provision of some form of parenting support, or a clinical intervention, such as a decision about a drug or a surgical procedure, is faced with a formidable task. The research findings to help answer the question may well exist, but locating that research, assessing its evidential 'weight' and relevance and incorporating it into other information is often difficult.

The systematic review is a method of critically appraising, summarising and attempting to reconcile the evidence about a particular question (Petticrew and Roberts, 2006). The value of systematic reviews is that they provide a synthesis of robust studies in a particular field of work which no practitioner, however diligent, could possibly hope to read themselves at the same time as doing their day job. Systematic reviews are an important means of pulling together a range of research evidence. They are neither new nor particularly medical, and literature reviews are a core part of all academic fields. What is more recent, is the emphasis on the potential for systematic reviews to inform social policy decision making. One of the main differences between systematic and other literature reviews lies in the strong emphasis in the former on limiting bias, on attempting to locate *all* the relevant evidence, and on basing the review conclusions only on the best available evidence once the included studies have been critically appraised.

Systematic reviews have often been mischaracterised as being grand summaries which ignore modifiers of effectiveness. However, they can rigorously assess 'what works for whom' by exploring similarities and differences between studies and groups of studies; in fact the assessment of heterogeneity is one of the important elements of any systematic review.

Good examples of evidence syntheses which use systematic reviews, maps and other methods that consider contextual information are those produced by the EPPI-Centre at the Institute of Education, University of London. The combinations of methods they use, and their syntheses of trial results and users' views have particular potential for exploring inequalities in health and what to do about them (Oliver et al., 2006). One example of such a process is provided by Rees et al. (2006) in their study of young people and physical activity (see Figure 2.1).

Systematic reviews differ from traditional narrative reviews in a number of ways:

- The objectives of the review are specified.
- The materials and methods used are specified in advance, for example, the criteria for inclusion or exclusion of studies.
- They seek to identify and review all relevant studies.
- They assess the methodological soundness of the studies they include.
- The review can be replicated by others addressing the same question using the same materials and methods.

Figure 2.1: The review process: young people and physical activity

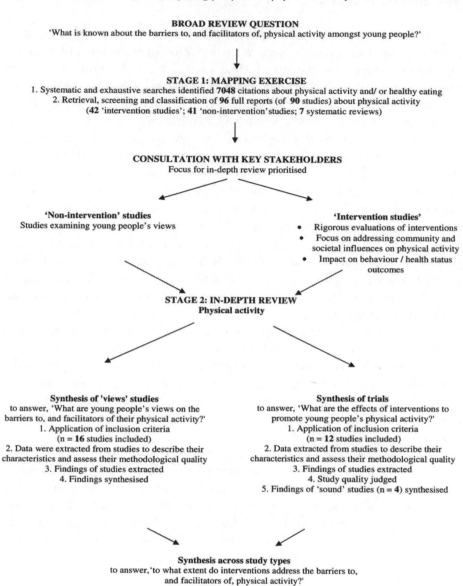

BROAD REVIEW QUESTION
'What is known about the barriers to, and facilitators of, physical activity amongst young people?'

STAGE 1: MAPPING EXERCISE
1. Systematic and exhaustive searches identified **7048** citations about physical activity and/ or healthy eating
2. Retrieval, screening and classification of **96** full reports (of **90** studies) about physical activity
(**42** 'intervention studies'; **41** 'non-intervention' studies; **7** systematic reviews)

CONSULTATION WITH KEY STAKEHOLDERS
Focus for in-depth review prioritised

'Non-intervention' studies
Studies examining young people's views

'Intervention studies'
- Rigorous evaluations of interventions
- Focus on addressing community and societal influences on physical activity
- Impact on behaviour / health status outcomes

STAGE 2: IN-DEPTH REVIEW
Physical activity

Synthesis of 'views' studies
to answer, 'What are young people's views on the barriers to, and facilitators of their physical activity?'
1. Application of inclusion criteria
(n = **16** studies included)
2. Data were extracted from studies to describe their characteristics and assess their methodological quality
3. Findings of studies extracted
4. Findings synthesised

Synthesis of trials
to answer, 'What are the effects of interventions to promote young people's physical activity?'
1. Application of inclusion criteria
(n = **12** studies included)
2. Data extracted from studies to describe their characteristics and assess their methodological quality
3. Findings of studies extracted
4. Study quality judged
5. Findings of 'sound' studies (n = **4**) synthesised

Synthesis across study types
to answer, 'to what extent do interventions address the barriers to, and facilitators of, physical activity?'

Reprinted with permission from Oxford University Press; from Rees, R., Kavanagh, J., Harden, A., Shepherd, J., Brunton, G., Oliver, S. and Oakley, A. 'Young people and physical activity: a systematic review matching their views to effective interventions', *Health Education Research*, 2006, 21(6): pp 806-25

Systematic reviews are thus unlike 'reviews of the studies I could find', 'reviews of the authors I admire', 'reviews which leave out inconveniently inconclusive findings or findings I don't like' and 'reviews which support the policy or intervention I intend to introduce'. They are more reliable than other kinds of reviews as they critically appraise the studies they include, and are based on the most methodologically sound research. They are sometimes characterised as too narrow to be helpful outside clinical medicine, or as being restricted to RCTs. However, good systematic reviews do not exclude any study design relevant to the question asked. As Petticrew (2001) points out, systematic reviews have been used not just to answer 'Does Drug A work better than Drug B?' but also a wide range of non-clinical questions ranging from: 'Are jurors influenced by the defendant's race?' (Sweeney and Haney, 1992) to 'Does the sexual orientation of parents matter in terms of parenting style, emotional adjustment or sexual orientation of children?' (Allen and Burrell, 1996).

Other good sources of reviews touching on inequalities in health include those from the Cochrane Public Health Group which facilitates the production of systematic reviews of the effects of public health interventions to improve health and other outcomes *at the population level*, rather than those targeted at individuals. Thus, it covers interventions seeking to address the broad determinants of health. Interventions in this field are often multi-sectoral, that is, not confined just to those developed and delivered within the health sector. Topics include welfare to work interventions and their effects on the health and well-being of lone parents and their children, and later school start times for supporting the education, health and well-being of those at secondary school.

Another important source in this context is a published protocol for a review of knowledge translation strategies for facilitating evidence-informed public health decision making among managers and policy makers (Armstrong et al., 2011). Further good sources for evidence in this field are the Campbell Collaboration, The Centre for Excellence and Outcomess in Children's and Young People's Services (C4EO) and NHS Evidence.

Demonstrating that systematic reviews are not all about trials, the box below describes a suite of studies on childhood obesity published by the EPPI-Centre.

Childhood obesity

There is considerable policy interest in the UK and internationally in tackling overweight and obesity in children and young people. However, no one review can hope to answer all the questions that policy makers or programme managers might have. The EPPI-Centre's studies summarised here can be sourced through the web link.

Children's views

This review examined research findings from the UK, where children aged 4 to 11 provided views about their body size or the body size of others. Many were dissatisfied and some felt anxious despite having a healthy body size. Fat-related name calling and bullying was considered to be a normal occurrence (Rees et al., 2009).

Sedentary behaviour

A systematic map reviewed studies on the relationship between obesity and sedentary behaviour in young people aged 6 to 16. The most frequent measure was time spent in TV, film and video viewing, followed by computer use/playing computer games/owning a computer and playing video games. The review found 197 studies that attempted to assess the effect of sedentary behaviour on obesity, 65 studies that aimed to assess the effect of obesity on sedentary behaviour, and eight studies that assessed both. In addition, 41 intervention studies attempted to manipulate sedentary behaviour and assess its effect on obesity (Kalra and Newman, 2009).

Educational attainment

Twenty-nine studies on the link between obesity and educational attainment were reviewed. The overall pattern suggested that heavier weight is associated with lower educational attainment. Place of residence, ethnicity, occupation, gender, religion, education, socioeconomic status and social capital were all explored. Most studies looked at the influence of obesity upon attainment; two examined the influence of attainment on obesity (Caird et al., 2011).

Social and environmental interventions

Interventions that aim to change social and environmental factors in order to reduce obesity may include taxes or subsidies to encourage healthy eating or physical activity; extra provision of sporting facilities; efforts to improve the safety and accessibility of walking and cycling or play areas; or attempting to influence the social meanings attached to weight, food or physical activity. A systematic map identified 54 reviews, of which 32 were systematic. Some focused on specific intervention strategies, such as point-of-sale information. Some investigated multi-component interventions which integrated social and environmental change with education and strategies for individual behaviour change, in either school or community settings. Few reviews were found which included studies evaluating large-scale structural changes to the physical environment or the availability or cost of food, exercise or sport (Woodman et al., 2008).

The use of incentives

A systematic map of studies which evaluated the use of incentives to tackle obesity, physical activity, diet and weight management behaviours found 61 studies, of which 20% included young people, 32% children and 17% the general population. Fifteen studies (25%) evaluated the use of incentives in low-income populations. A broad range of incentives was provided, with financial incentives being the most common (Kavanagh et al., 2009).

A database of schemes to promote healthy weight

The Department of Health (England) commissioned a report and associated searchable database to summarise schemes for promoting healthy weight in England. In order to be included in the database, schemes needed a primary focus on tackling overweight or obesity in school-age children who were already overweight or obese. Included interventions had to be structured and sustained over a period of time. The data covered the content and running of the scheme, as well as noting any monitoring or evaluation that had taken place (Aicken et al., 2008).

Summarised from the EPPI-Centre website, http://eppi.ioe.ac.uk/cms/Default.aspx?tabid=2957

The contribution of different research designs

Lessons to be learned from large-scale evaluations

The majority of robustly evaluated early childhood initiatives were launched in the US (Oakley, 1998, 2000), with at least 30 federal educational and training programmes for low-income populations in the 1960s and 1970s (Levin, 1978). A major objective was to increase the basic cognitive skills of disadvantaged children, so there was a good deal of emphasis on measured IQ as an outcome. However, some programmes took a broader view of the positive outcomes which might be encouraged by early intervention. Many other large-scale evaluations of social programmes were launched in the US covering such fields as income maintenance, and training and employment initiatives for socially disadvantaged groups (Boruch and Riecken, 1975). These raised a number of points about both effective evaluation and effective implementation, including:

- the need to take into account the complexity of social settings;
- involving the 'targets' of intervention in designing appropriate initiatives and outcomes;
- distinguishing between individuals, families, households and communities as targets of intervention; and
- the importance of a multi-disciplinary approach to evaluation.

Design problems characteristic of the early intervention field (Farran, 1990; Gallagher, 1990; Hauser-Cram, 1990) include:

- lack of standardisation of the intervention, leading to unmanageable variability between sites;
- narrow outcome measures; and
- lack of comparability between intervention and control groups, leading to probable underestimates of social programme effectiveness.

An important programme in the UK has been Sure Start, where there was strong prima facie evidence that what was being offered to children seemed likely, on the basis of strong research evidence, to make a positive difference (Glass, 1999; Roberts, 2000). Unfortunately the evaluation has not been able to demonstrate the outcomes expected. The evaluators reported a quasi-experimental cross-sectional study on the effects of Sure Start local programmes (SSLPs) on children and their families, attempting to assess whether variations in the effectiveness of SSLPs were due to differences in implementation (Belsky et al., 2006). The settings were 150 socially deprived communities in England with ongoing SSLPs and 50 comparison communities. The outcome measures were mothers' reports of community services and their local areas, family functioning and parenting skills, child health and development, and verbal ability at 36 months. What they found was that SSLPs seem to benefit relatively less socially deprived parents (who may have greater personal resources) and their children, but seem to have an adverse effect on the most disadvantaged children. Programmes led by health services seem to be more effective than programmes led by other agencies.

As the evaluators pointed out in a further report, (NESS team, 2010) they faced a number of methodological challenges, including early decisions not to undertake an RCT, and a doubling in the number of SLPs early on, reducing the opportunity to identify suitable comparison areas.

Surveys

The survey is a not a method which lends itself to answering the question 'what works?' but it would be difficult for managers or commissioners of services to plan without good data on the scale of particular problems, and what users think about problems and interventions. Well-designed surveys can provide useful information about prevalence; poor surveys, on the other hand, can exacerbate problems, as in the case of surveys of incidence and prevalence which use vague definitions. Rates of child sexual abuse, for instance, an important problem, have been estimated by various studies as being between 3% and 90% (Pilkington and Kremer, 1995).

Surveys can also provide powerful descriptive feedback following policy changes or widespread new service provision, as the next box demonstrates.

A survey of parents in the areas covered by Sure Start in 2008 (TNS, 2009), designed to quantify awareness and use of the centre found that the reach of children's centres was good with 78% of parents and carers aware of their local centre and 45% having used it. The profile of centre users was very similar to the profile of respondents, suggesting that reach was good throughout the target population. Childcare and nursery education were the most heavily used services at the centres and at the time of the survey, one quarter of the respondents were currently using them. Use of health services and family and parenting services was less widespread – 13% of respondents had used health services in the three months prior to the survey and 9% had used family and parenting services. Finally, those who had used or attended their local centre were very happy with the services they had used. When considering all of the services they had used at the centre, 92% of users said they were satisfied and of these, 68% were very satisfied. Knowing which services people opt into (and which they drop out of) is important data for those providing them.

Surveys can also shed light on the gaps that can exist between the good intentions behind organisational and policy changes and the working reality. This can help explore reasons why things might not be working according to plan. In terms of advocacy, surveys can also be a useful way to grab the headlines – though as with all interventions, there may be unforeseen negative consequences, as described in the next box.

A survey with unforeseen consequences

A survey which had interesting (and possibly useful) findings (Reinisch and Sanders, 1999) also had an unexpected negative consequence for the editor of the *Journal of the American Medical Association* (*JAMA*). Based on data from a 1991 survey of 599 students at a large mid-Western university, it indicated that American university students did not consider that oral sex counted as having sex. 'The current public debate regarding whether oral sex constitutes having "had sex" or sexual relations has suffered from a lack of empirical data on how Americans as a population define these terms,' the authors wrote. Their survey showed that 60% of students did not consider oral-genital sex to be real sex: 'almost everyone agreed that penile-vaginal intercourse would qualify as having "had sex" ' (Tanne, 1999). The publication coincided with the impeachment of President Clinton on charges of perjury in relation to sexual activity. The editor of *JAMA* was dismissed because he had fast-tracked the publication. A statement explaining the dismissal claimed that the editor had threatened the integrity of *JAMA* by 'inexcusably interjecting [the American Medical Association] into a major political debate that has nothing to do with science or medicine'.

The cohort studies

Probably the best sources of data on a statistical association between early childhood events and later outcomes are the cohort studies. These collect both health and social data at intervals, often from shortly after birth until well into adulthood. Data are collected from the same people over a period of years, so that information on a child at, say, one, five or nine years old, can be related to the same child (now adult) at 19 or 29 or 49 years. From the cohort studies, we know that risks of death and serious illness are greatest for those brought up in the lowest socioeconomic groups (Power et al., 1991; Wadsworth, 1991; Power and Hertzman, 1997; Hawkes et al., 2004; Dex and Joshi, 2005).

Although, over a period of time, some people become lost to follow-up, data from these studies remain a remarkable repository of information on the growth and development of children and young people. As the cohorts progress into adulthood, they allow researchers to explore associations between early childhood experiences and later characteristics. Thus the cohort studies can enable us to identify factors which seem to have a protective effect. In other words they can help us understand why some children, given a poor start in life, do well. Identifying factors which seem to have made a difference to the children who have overcome the disadvantages of their early years is the first step in identifying what might be done to help children to overcome adverse circumstances. The question of exactly *what* is making the difference is a question for these, as for other sources of data. The 'cohort effect' – the fact that this is a group of children and young people born and growing up in a particular era and social and economic framework, has to be considered in assessing the results.

Some of the cohort studies, for which the UK has a strong reputation, are described below. Of particular relevance to children and families are the birth cohort studies in which those included are selected into the study at birth and followed up at intervals. Such studies produce a wealth of data, becoming more useful as the children get older – hence the importance of long-term follow-up into adulthood.

Some of the key studies have generated many publications, of which examples include:

- The National Survey of Health and Development (Wadsworth, 1991; Kuh et al., 2009)
- The National Child Development Study (Ferri, 1993; Elliott, 2008)
- Newcastle Thousand Families Study (Kolvin et al.,1983; Wright et al., 2001)
- Aberdeen Child Development Study (Illsley, 1967; Hagger-Johnson et al., 2011)
- Child Health and Education Study (re-named in 1991 the British Cohort Study 1970) (Osborn and Milbank,1985; Bynner and Joshi, 2002)
- Avon Longitudinal Study of Parents and Children (ALSPAC) (Golding et al., 1992; Barker et al., 2011)
- Twenty-07 study (Sweeting and West, 1995; Benzeval et al., 2009)
- The Millennium Cohort (Dex and Joshi, 2005; Bartington et al., 2006)

A new Birth Cohort Study (BCS), beginning in or around 2013 will track the growth, development, health, well-being and social circumstances of over 90,000 UK babies and their families from all walks of life and will initially cover the period from pregnancy right through the early years of childhood. Key areas of enquiry include charting the social diversity of the next generation of UK citizens, including income, poverty and inequalities, family structure, ethnic identities and intergenerational social mobility; educational research on antecedents of school readiness and educational performance; and interplay between key health and other outcomes. A new Cohort Resources Facility will integrate data from new and existing cohort studies.

The cohort studies can give an indication of the effects of changing social and family policies, as well as the effects of particular ways of living family life. Ferri (1993:3–4) asked: 'the moves towards ameliorating economic and social inequality, which took place during the childhood of the National Child Development Study sample have been reversed in recent years ... What have all these changes meant for the lives and experiences of those in their thirties?' It would be misleading to suggest that the cohort studies can give complete answers to questions about what works in family and social policies, but they provide important pointers, sufficiently so to have attracted almost £30 million in funding for the new BCS at a time of some austerity in the UK.

Randomised controlled trials

The strongest research design in attributing a particular result to a particular intervention is the RCT. Random allocation reduces the risk of bias from important unmeasured as well as measured confounding factors, which might otherwise lead us astray. If we are interested in exploring whether *this* particular intervention has *that* particular effect, then RCTs provide the most compelling evidence. We may want to ask, for instance whether:

- a particular sex education programme reduces the rate of teenage pregnancies;
- providing an income supplement for pregnant women at risk of a low birthweight baby leads to heavier babies;
- exercise programmes for young people can reduce the number of cigarettes they smoke.

In these cases, an RCT will provide us with good evidence of a causal relationship between an intervention and an outcome. The best evidence will come from a number of trials, synthesised in a systematic review.

RCTs are studies in which one group (the experimental group) receives a particular intervention and another group (the control group) receives a different intervention or none at all. True randomisation can only be said to have occurred where all clients have an equal chance of being allocated to either group. Any bias, for example by allocating certain clients to the experimental group because they are likely to 'do better', invalidates findings, as randomisation is not carried out by those delivering the intervention.

RCTs do not remove all our problems; for example, we may well worry about what our 'intervention' actually is. If work with a group is effective, is its effectiveness due to the discussions, the workers' directions or the companionship of others? We need to ensure that the measures we use are meaningful, and that the changes reported are not due to bias in those gathering the information. These are problems we have to address whatever our research design. But because randomisation abolishes selection biases, it can help to settle disputes about the relative efficacy of two forms of intervention, or of intervention versus non-intervention.

People worry about the ethics of randomisation, particularly randomisation to 'no treatment', and others, including one of the paediatricians who worked on the causes of a form of blindness seen in premature babies, have highlighted the lengths to which people will go to subvert the randomisation process, because of concerns about client welfare (Silverman, 1980). The starting point for randomisation however, is that we frequently do not know what works, or what works best. In the experiment described by Silverman, the findings suggested that the intervention into which so many professionals were so keen to enter babies may have been harmful. Well-run trials have independent data and safety monitoring boards whose role is to try to ensure that if the data show that continuing the trial will do harm (either by exposing people to a harmful intervention or denying them an intervention where the treatment effects are strongly positive, it is terminated early. As Jensen and Hampton (2007) point out, data and safety monitoring boards tread a delicate path. Patients in a trial should not be exposed to undue risks, but if a trial is stopped without compelling evidence of benefit or harm, people may later be denied potentially helpful treatments. Indeed, it has been suggested that stopping a trial with harmful events may not be without harm to participants, and can be experienced as denying hope to participants who have seen the intervention as a last chance. A rapid response to the Jensen and Hampton article describes a study (Coleman, 2005) where the authors outline the distress of participants in a multiple sclerosis treatment trial when it was terminated early, concluding: 'Members of such boards can take little comfort from our observation that apparent understanding by research subjects at the outset that a clinical drug trial may be terminated, does not ensure acceptance of this as an outcome.'[1] The longer the follow-up from an RCT the more useful the evidence is likely to be. Most weight management interventions for children, for instance, are likely to result in weight loss in the short term, but longer-term follow-ups are rare. In the Perry High/Scope study described in Chapter Three, the positive effects of the intervention in terms of school readiness appeared to wear off at age seven. It was only later that many other positive effects of the intervention were measured and described.

Studies with quasi-experimental designs

The realities of services for children mean that it is not always possible to randomly allocate children and families to different services or control groups derived from waiting lists. What is essential is that alternative approaches to evaluation are designed, analysed and interpreted in ways that maximise our knowledge of the relationship between what we do and any changes seen. A method more commonly used than RCTs is to design studies that have one or more control groups, but no random allocation. These are quasi-experimental studies.

These studies are similar to RCTs insofar as some clients receive a service, while others do not, or receive a different service. But instead of random allocation, researchers take clients occurring 'naturally', and establish a control group matched on characteristics thought to be important, for example, socioeconomic status, severity of problem, duration of problem and so on. This might happen where a team in one area favours one approach, a team in another area a different approach. The trouble is that it is impossible to match in a way which takes account of all relevant factors, known and unknown. Only randomisation can do this. While the study in the box that follows has promising findings, and unlike the Sure Start evaluation, has the advantage of pre-intervention data, the authors acknowledge that for a study of this kind, an RCT would have been the optimal design.

---

[1] www.bmj.com/content/334/7589/326?tab=responses

Example of a quasi-experimental design

Communities for Children (CfC) is part of the Australian Family Support Programme, which provides prevention and early intervention programmes to families with children up to 12 years at risk of disadvantage and disconnected from childhood services. A quasi-experimental cohort study in socioeconomically disadvantaged communities evaluated the early effects of CfC and whether the effectiveness differed for less-advantaged families.

Outcome measures included child health and development, family functioning and parenting. After controlling for background factors, there were beneficial effects associated with CfC, showing some benefits for child receptive vocabulary, parenting and reducing jobless households. Children living in the most disadvantaged households were reported to benefit.

Edwards et al. (2011)

Evaluation studies with non-experimental designs

Research designs within this category are evaluated interventions but with no random allocation and no pre-intervention matching of groups, if indeed a comparison group is used at all. Taken singly, results based on studies using these designs are, at best, only suggestive. However, confidence can be enhanced in two ways. Firstly, if a number of such studies featuring a range of clients in different circumstances produce similar results, one can feel more confident that the intervention may be influencing the changes. Such a pattern would indicate that it might be worth investing the time and resources involved in experimental research to place these results on a more secure footing. Secondly, if experimental studies featuring similar procedures and approaches already exist, we can have more confidence in interpreting the results of non-experimental studies.

In order to evaluate a service, it is important to know what outcomes we are trying to achieve and how we are hoping to achieve them, and to have before and after measures. If things are not working as well as they might, we need to understand why not. Using a theory of change (Connell and Kubisch, 1998) can help with this, as can using a logic model (see University of Wisconsin, 2002–5).

Qualitative research

The development of effective services also requires other kinds of evidence. Some of the most important research questions are those which are addressed by qualitative research. These are the questions which enable us to know whether a particular intervention is salient for the people to whom it is offered, and what they consider the important outcomes to be. Those on the receiving end of health or welfare services have a reservoir of expertise on their own lives.

Without qualitative studies, we would be hard pressed to understand the social worlds of those living with inequality, and without this understanding, we cannot begin to conceptualise interventions which will be acceptable, let alone effective. The research designs we describe earlier are those which cast light on the relationship between what we do and changes experienced by those with whom we work. The confidence we can have that a particular set of outcomes is attributable to our actions depends in large part on the research design and its careful execution.

Qualitative research carried out prior to RCTs for instance, and then incorporated into the process of running trials, can help to identify which interventions and outcomes are most likely to be important, and how particular interventions should be delivered. Death in a house fire has the steepest social class gradient of any cause of death in childhood. Qualitative research with children and adults run in tandem with an RCT in inner city London helped to identify why smoke alarms designed to prevent a fire taking hold are disabled; what children do when they hear a domestic smoke alarm go off and why some adults disable their alarms or prefer not to have them installed (Rowland et al., 2002; Roberts et al., 2004a).

User views

Users want to have services which make a difference. Their life experience may mean that they are better able than some professionals to accept that some things work better than others, and that not everything helps. Providing services which are likely to benefit users (and unlikely to harm them) requires their involvement in the planning, development and monitoring of those services. Powerful though not uncritical alliances have been forged, for instance, between young people with disabilities and those who provide services, women having babies and birth attendants, and looked-after children and care leavers and policy makers. Each is in a position to draw on the expertise of the other, although the alliances themselves, and their outcomes, positive and negative, also need to be evaluated.

A gap between research evidence and the views of those who use services (or more often, a gap between those who provide services and those who decline to use them, or use them once but never again) may raise serious questions about the intervention. A variety of methods have been suggested to overcome this, including devising outcome measures in consultation with clients or users. In some cases, interventions may be justified on the basis of positive client accounts alone, especially where no harmful effects are likely and the views of all clients involved in the programme are solicited. Equally, however, regarding clients' views on the effectiveness of an intervention as the sole criterion for judging success ignores a substantial body of evidence on the poor correlation between the strength of client approval and the impact of the intervention when considered by third parties (Macdonald et al., 1992). The 'fit' between satisfaction (or dissatisfaction) with a service and the achievement of the desired outcome is not as good as it might be (McCord, 1981). Users of services frequently like the people providing the service, and are grateful. They may be concerned that criticism may deprive them of any service at all. This does not always mean that they are getting the most effective service that they could.

User studies are nonetheless an important source of data, and one in which the British have a good track record. Work with children as primary respondents was until recently under-developed. The techniques and methods for involving children and young people have greatly improved over the last two decades, as has attention to ethical issues including consent (Alderson and Morrow, 2011). Our capacity to consult children, including marginalised children, is better than it was. Methodological problems remain, however. Children, no less than adults, frequently want to please. The lesson from this is that good interviewing involves building relationships (Oakley, 1981). 'Spray on' focus group consultations may provide good sound-bites, but are unlikely to produce sound evidence. However, spray on messages may convey their own powerful dispatches from frontline users. The image in Figure 2.2, 'Help I'm ill', although hardly a research finding, is one that resulted in remarkably speedy change. The author happened to see this in a local street on the way to present findings from a review of children's views of local services. While the recommendations of the report itself took the usual course of discussion followed by modest action over a period of some years, this did not happen rapidly. However, showing the picture had a much more dramatic effect. By the following week, the message had disappeared from the newly painted shutters completely. Cosmetic changes can be enacted more speedily than service changes.

An assets-based approach drawing on lay and scientific evidence

Many projects with minority ethnic families aim to act on individual and family behaviour – making 'them' more like 'us' rather than learning from their strengths, and tackling the issues which may make services less than welcoming, or inappropriate. Described below is a refreshing project in progress which aims to work with the cultural competence of those delivering services as well as learning from those who receive (or avoid) those services.

There is a steep social class gradient in dental caries, and as Watt (2007) has pointed out, the dominant method of dealing with this has been through narrowly focused 'lifestyle' interventions which fail to address the underlying social determinants of health inequalities and are 'victim-blaming' in nature.

Figure 2.2: 'Help I'm ill'

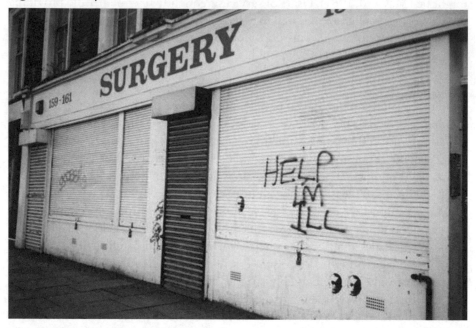

Reprinted with permission from BMJ Publishing Group; from Roberts, H. 'Help I'm Ill', *Journal of Epidemiology and Community Health*, 2008, 62:572

Teeth Tales: understanding the issues

In a piece of work consistent with this model, and working in partnership with the community in Victoria, Australia, Teeth Tales has used qualitative research methods to explore the social, cultural and environmental determinants of the development of poor child oral health in refugee and migrant communities. Mothers and grandmothers from Iraqi (Assyrian Chaldean), Pakistani and Lebanese communities participated in focus groups and interviews involving community leaders, parents and grandparents. Dental and other health professionals were also interviewed.

Findings were integrated with existing evidence on effective interventions, using socio-environmental models of health to develop a culturally competent community-based oral health research intervention and evaluation plan, with solutions identified by the community informing the intervention which has been developed to form the second phase of Teeth Tales.

Among the elements addressed, services and programmes provided by community health services and local governments will take part in a review in order to identify organisational strengths in cultural competency and areas for improvement. They will then be assisted to progress their organisation to become culturally competent at all organisational levels (Gibbs et al., 2009).

www.mccaugheycentre.unimelb.edu.au/research/current/intergenerational_health/teeth_tales

Figure 2.3 demonstrates the different levels at which poor dental health might be tackled, ranging from the clinical to the population-based. While each level may have its strengths, it is by acting on the causes of the causes that we are likely to see inequalities narrowed.

Figure 2.3: Upstream/downstream: options for oral disease prevention

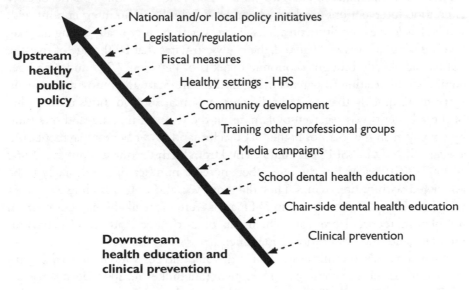

Costs and cost-effectiveness

Evidence-informed policy and practice also needs to address the costs and benefits of particular interventions and the ways in which services are organised and delivered. The modern child in western societies is both economically inefficient and emotionally priceless (Zelizer, 1994). However, while the rhetoric of investing in children in the UK has placed an emphasis on the value of children and the value of families, the impetus for action probably owes more to the well-crafted US trials of early childhood interventions in which children have been followed up well into adulthood (eg Schweinhart and Weikart, 1997). Work from the US suggesting that for every $1 spent, $7 was saved, elicited particular interest in the UK from both the Treasury and the Home Office. While metrics showing what can be saved by spending now may well have lost some traction as an advocacy tool through overuse, it is important to know more about what is cost-effective, as well as what is effective.

This suggests that greater investment needs to be made in building the research evidence base on the cost-effectiveness of non-clinical interventions in the early years, childhood, adolescence and young adulthood. This needs to take into account a wide range of outcomes of importance to children and parents, service providers and policy makers, and of what is most likely to affect long-term outcomes and benefits not only to children and adolescents themselves, but to the entire community. As Meadows (2010) has pointed out in an economic perspective on the National Evaluation of Sure Start (NESS), the economic benefits of early childhood interventions can be high (and much higher than interventions with similar levels of expenditure on adults). However, there is typically a long time lag before savings are made. That said, the study estimates that by the age of five, the SSLPs had already brought economic benefits of between £279 and £557 per eligible child, relating to parents living in the Sure Start areas moving into paid work more quickly than those in the comparison areas. Two thirds of the value of these benefits was received by families in the form of income, and one third by tax payers in the form of higher tax receipts and lower benefit payments. On average, the cost of SSLPs per eligible child from birth to four was put at £4,860 at 2009–2010 prices, but the researchers noted a number of trends likely to be associated with future savings. They did, however, also note a finding associated with later costs. Mothers living in SSLP areas were more likely than comparison mothers to report depression, which can be associated with child behaviour problems and lower educational attainment.

Discussions of economic evaluation in this area and costs and benefits built into evaluations are now becoming more frequent (Shemilt et al., 2004; Beecham et al., 2007; Stevens et al., 2010) with creative theoretical work in relation to complex interventions (Shiell et al., 2008).

What doesn't work?

There are a number of barriers to our learning about what doesn't work. We know that there are publication biases, with researchers more ready to submit articles with 'positive' results, and journals more ready to accept these for publication. In addition, there are strong disincentives to describing what goes wrong in funded projects. 'Will I look incompetent?' 'What will the funders think?' 'I shouldn't have allowed that to happen' (Bell and Newby, 1977; Bell and Roberts, 1984). Presentations at large conferences almost always have a positive spin, so that other practitioners, trying to replicate what sounded like a perfectly formed, simple intervention with a large effect size may become downhearted when life isn't quite like that.

Government policy is not free from building on what does not work. Extensive evaluation has suggested that the 'Scared Straight' (see following box) experiments tried in the US with young offenders have had the reverse of the desired effect (Utting and Vennard, 2000; Petrosino et al., 2002). This has not prevented 'tough measures' with young offenders being called for by the popular press and proposed by successive UK home secretaries.

Scared Straight

'Scared Straight' and other programmes involve organised visits to prison by juvenile delinquents or children 'at risk' of criminal behaviour. These visits are intended to deter participants from future offending through first-hand observation of prison life and meeting adult inmates. They remain in use despite studies and reviews questioning their effectiveness.

In a systematic review of trials, Petrosino et al. (2002) showed the intervention to be more harmful than doing nothing. The authors conclude that programmes like 'Scared Straight' are likely to have a harmful effect and increase delinquency relative to doing nothing at all with the same young people. The authors caution: 'Given these results, agencies that permit such programmes must rigorously evaluate them not only to ensure that they are doing what they purport to do (prevent crime) – but at the very least they do not cause more harm than good'.

In aviation and anaesthetics, there are procedures (imperfect though they sometimes are), for reviewing both where things have gone wrong, and where near-mistakes have been noticed and disaster averted. We need to encourage a culture where as researchers and practitioners, we can learn from mistakes as well as from successes.

Making it work

Knowing that an intervention works is no guarantee that it will be used, no matter how obvious or simple it is to implement. For example, it is nearly 150 years since Semmelweis's trial showed that handwashing reduces infection, yet health care workers' compliance with handwashing remains poor (Teare et al., 2001). Even the most simple, cost-effective and logical intervention fails if people will not carry it out (Sheldon et al., 1998). An RCT, well conducted, can tell us which kind of smoke alarm is most likely to be functioning 18 months after installation, but it cannot tell us what the best way is to work effectively with housing managers to make sure alarms are installed effectively and cost-effectively, while also ensuring that the households of the most vulnerable tenants are included.

The obstacles and levers for the uptake of research findings are likely to be understood through methods different from those usually found at the top of traditional hierarchies of evidence (Halladay and Bero, 2000; Nutley et al., 2007). It may therefore be most useful to think about how to best use the wide range of evidence available – and particularly to consider what types of study are most suitable for answering particular types of question.

In many cases, the most important outcomes of the interventions in childhood are not known for many years, and it may be difficult to distinguish the effects of our interventions from maturational effects – that is, children and young people change as they grow up. It is also important to recall, as set out earlier, that no evidence of effect is not the same as evidence of no effect. Many promising programmes have not been evaluated with long enough follow-up times to know whether positive (or negative) outcomes are temporary or longer lasting.

Key messages

- As in every other field of human endeavour, some things work better than others.
- Not all research helps us understand what works. Knowing what users, politicians or professionals think about a service doesn't help us know how *effective* it is.
- Without lay expertise, however effective a service intervention is, it may not be used.
- There is no hierarchy of evidence – different research methods are needed to answer different kinds of question.
- In times of austerity, it becomes particularly important to spend on services which bring about improvements and are acceptable (and preferably enjoyable) to those who use them.
- A first step in thinking about designing interventions for children is to find, commission or conduct a systematic review. What do we already know from well-conducted studies about intervening in this particular problem? How can we use what we know?

THREE

What works in early life? Infancy and the pre-school period

Investment in the early years provides one of the greatest potentials to reduce health inequities within a generation. Experiences in early childhood (defined as prenatal development to eight years of age), and in early and later education, lay critical foundations for the entire life course (Irwin et al., 2007).

The best time to intervene to reduce health inequalities now and in the future is in early life, although the recent enthusiasm for early years' interventions should not lead anyone to suppose that it is ever too late to change the course of a child's or young person's life. An understanding of the importance of early interventions and of the determinants of good health in the under-fives, informed and supported by good evidence, is the foundation for policies to promote child health.

Changes for the better in early child health
- Death in infancy and childhood is rare in the UK.
- Many more children now have the benefit of good-quality care in childhood as a result of high-quality programmes such as Sure Start (now Sure Start Children's Centres).

But inequality remains a problem
- Children born into poverty are more likely to be born early or born small.
- These children have elevated health risks (Macfarlane and Mugford, 2000).
- For babies whose fathers have a routine or manual occupation, the mortality rate in 2004–06 was 17% higher than that for the general population, compared to 13% higher in 1997–99 (Department of Health, 2008).
- In England and Wales in 2005 and 2006, babies in the Caribbean and Pakistani ethnic groups were more than twice as likely to die before the age of one than babies from the White British population (Hollowell et al., 2011).
- While mortality has markedly decreased over the last century, reported ill health among children is rising, with particular increases in respiratory diseases, including asthma, and emotional problems (Prescott-Clarke and Primatesta, 1998).

If intervening in the early years is as powerful as we believe, we need to be as certain as we can that when we intervene in the lives of children, there is evidence that our interventions will do some good. This chapter describes, with examples, some of the practice interventions which make a difference. In evaluating for effectiveness, there are some interventions in people's lives that we can take for granted are a good thing. A roof over your head and enough to eat are not interventions that need to be tested through a randomised controlled trial (RCT), though what constitutes a 'good diet', and how best to ensure that housing and adequate nutrition are delivered is susceptible to investigation.

There is, of course, no magic bullet, and looking to other countries for evidence of 'what works' and using these to identify single interventions or policies will be nugatory unless we look at the whole package of income, childcare, family support, schooling, housing and the way that children and parents are valued. It is important to remember that what works in one country and at one time cannot automatically be applied with the same success somewhere else and in different circumstances. While certain kinds of research evidence, particularly trial evidence, are strong in the US, policy makers also need to look closer to home, in particular to the Nordic countries, if we are to pursue policies and practices which will help create a fairer society in which children can thrive. In Chapter Seven, Figure 7.1, based on UNICEF's reports on of child well-being, shows children in Finland, Norway, Denmark and Sweden all doing well, and the US, (from where many of our policy ideas are derived) an outlier doing rather badly.

Inequalities in health start early, at or even before birth. Poor parents are at greater risk of a stillborn baby, and babies born to poor parents are more likely to die in the first week of life (neonatal deaths) and the first year of life (infant deaths). They are more likely to be born early and born small. Even in countries with good obstetric and neonatal care, babies born early, and babies born small are at risk of a range of poor outcomes both in infancy and in later life.

There have been huge improvements in important measures of child health in high- and middle-income countries over the last century, although the UK is still rather poorly placed in the European league table of infant mortality. In 2004, the lowest infant mortality rates were to be found in Norway and Sweden, at 3 per thousand live births; the highest rate was in Latvia, at 9.4 per thousand live births. England and Wales and Scotland, all at 4.9 per thousand live births, are in the joint 20th place of 28 countries (Kurinczuk et al., 2009). An infant mortality rate of 6.9 per thousand in the US (World Bank, 2011) supports the view that it may be more useful to look towards northern Europe than towards the US, to which we frequently turn for examples of welfare policies associated with improvements in child health.

Important recent work on early life and health across the life course relies on medical records going back to the early part of the twentieth century in Hertfordshire, Preston and Sheffield. Using these, researchers have been able to show not only that poverty during foetal development and childhood affects health in the early years, but that it also adds to the burden of disease and premature death later (Barker, 1994). The early years are the foundation on which the rest of life is built.

Death in and before the first year

The context into which children are born in the UK, with free medical treatment at the point of need, is, of course, far more favourable than circumstances in most parts of the world. While at a global level, 98% of stillbirths occur in low- and middle-income countries, even in high-income countries, around 1 in every 320 babies is stillborn, and women from poorer backgrounds experience stillbirth far in excess of better-off women (Flenady et al., 2011). Deaths around the time of birth are normally linked to events during pregnancy and delivery and the care given to mothers and babies (Kurinczuk et al., 2009). Access to neonatal intensive care units blunts the effects of deprivation on infant death in very preterm infants, so as Gray and McCormick (2009) point out, achieving equitable outcomes requires medical care to be equally available and equally good across all settings. A study by Smith et al. (2009) looking at socioeconomic differences in survival rates and neonatal provision for very preterm babies in the UK found that such infants from deprived areas and those from affluent areas of the same gestational age and birthweight have similar levels of expected mortality and neonatal care. Deprivation does not seem to be a barrier to accessing and receiving neonatal care.

Demonstrating the importance of free access to the National Health Service (NHS) at the point of need, an example of what can happen when this is not the case is reported by Howell et al. (2008), who studied mortality differences in New York City. They found that White very low birthweight infants were more likely (49%) to be born in the third of hospitals with lowest mortality compared with Black very low birthweight infants (29%), and estimated that, if Black women delivered in the same hospitals as White women, 34.5% of the Black/White disparity in very low birthweight neonatal mortality rates in New York City would be removed.

Nevertheless, even in the UK with its NHS, those born into poverty are disadvantaged from (or even before) the start, with higher rates of stillbirth, maternal, neonatal and infant mortality among the poorest mothers and their children than among the better off. Table 3.1 sets out the definitions in relation to early deaths.

Infant mortality rates at or after 28 days have long been seen as an important indicator of population health (Kurinczuk et al., 2009), and deaths in early

Table 3.1: Infant death rates: definitions

Neonatal mortality rate (NNMR)	Deaths to babies under 28 days per 1,000 live births
Post-neonatal mortality rate (PNMR)	Deaths to babies aged 28 days and over and less than one year per 1,000 live births
Infant mortality rate (IMR)	Total deaths to infants under one year per 1,000 live births (comprising both neonatal and post-neonatal deaths)

childhood are frequently used as a proxy for a nation's general well-being. Poor survival in the early months indicates a society unable to protect the most vulnerable. Figure 3.1 shows the steady decline in infant mortality since the start of the 1980s. Within this, there is a gradient, with those in the poorest socioeconomic conditions and those registering a birth without a partner with the highest rates of death. These parents are also more likely to experience a child death through sudden infant death syndrome or the death of an infant from infection. There is a marked social class gradient, so it is not just the very poorest children whose health chances are affected by their circumstances. Less well-off children right across the board have poorer outcomes than those brought up in the most advantaged social circumstances (Gray et al., 2009). This gradient is also associated with lone motherhood and membership of a minority ethnic group, although as Figure 3.2 shows, not all minority ethnic groups have poorer outcomes.

Figure 3.1: Infant, neonatal and post-neonatal mortality rates, England and Wales 1980–2007

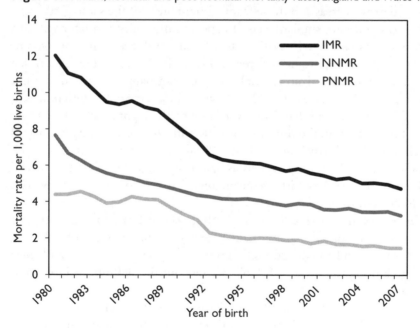

Note: For definitions, see Table 3.1.

Reprinted with permission from Inequalities in Infant Mortality, Project Briefing Paper 1 (Kurinczuk et al 2009) www.npeu.ox.ac.uk/infant-mortality

There are two main ways of measuring social inequalities in infant mortality (Gray et al., 2009): as a gradient across all groups, or as a gap between two groups. If interventions to tackle poor health are successful, it is possible to improve health overall while widening the gap.

This poses tricky ethical issues, discussed in 2006 at a three-day meeting on inequalities in health by the National Institute for Health and Clinical Excellence

Figure 3.2: Infant mortality by ethnic group, England and Wales 2005–06

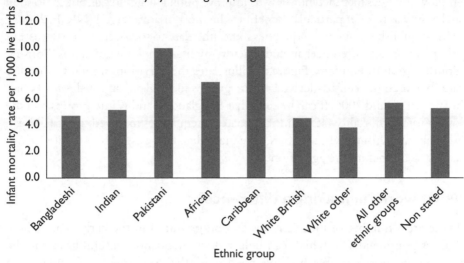

Reprinted with permission from W.B. Saunders Co.; from Hollowell, J., Kurinczuk, J., Brocklehurst, P. and Gray, R. 'Social and ethnic inequalities in infant mortality: a perspective from the United Kingdom', *Seminars in Perinatology*, 2011, vol 35 no 4, pp 240–4.

(NICE) Citizen's Council, a group of 30 people, all ordinary members of the public, who represented the make-up of the population of England and Wales. They were invited to think about which of two broad strategies it would be more appropriate for NICE to follow:

• whether to issue guidance that concentrates resources on improving the health of the whole population (which may mean improvement for all groups) even if there is a risk of widening the gap between socioeconomic groups;
• or whether to issue guidance that concentrates resources on trying to improve the health of the most disadvantaged members of society, thus narrowing the gap between the least and the most disadvantaged, even if this has only a modest impact on the health of the population as a whole.

Their view, despite many reservations, was that a narrow majority would look with sympathy on NICE strategies intended not only to improve public health for all, but to do so in a way that offers particular benefit to the most disadvantaged. In the final session, one council member referred to a passage from a Department of Health document she had looked up overnight reporting that babies born to poorer families are more likely to be born prematurely, are at greater risk of infant mortality, and have a greater likelihood of chronic disease in later life. The near unanimous view of the council was that they should be doing something about this. But in spite of the shared feeling about the unacceptability of the extremes of health inequality, a shared decision on how it should be tackled was not reached. However, they concluded that, where possible, the Institute should employ strategies intended not only to improve public health for all, but to do so in such a way as to offer particular benefit to the most disadvantaged (NICE, 2006a).

Most published data on inequalities in health relate to socioeconomic status, but other important differences include factors such as employment status, housing tenure, region or ethnicity. Figure 3.2 illustrates the variation in infant mortality rates between the census-derived ethnic groups in England and Wales for babies born in 2005 and 2006. It can be seen that Bangladeshi and White groups had the lowest infant mortality rates, and the greatest inequalities involved the Caribbean and Pakistani groups, whose babies were more than twice as likely as White British babies to die before the age of one.

What works in making a difference?

There are a number of interventions and programmes in the early years where there is good evidence which can help reduce inequalities in child health. The previous chapter describes how we need more than one source of evidence to enable effective services to be delivered. We need to know how big the problem is, what seems to be an effective way of dealing with it, what it costs, how it can be successfully delivered, and crucially, what those on the receiving end think about it. NICE, The Centre for Excellence and Outcomes in Children's and Young People's Services (C4EO) and NHS Evidence provide ready sources of evidence-informed support to decision makers, which includes not only the evidence, but also tools which can help with costs and implementation (see the Appendix).

Examples of interventions with the potential to reduce inequalities in child health for each chronological period are provided as follows.

In the ante-natal period

A range of protocols and guidelines, including the NICE guideline on intrapartum care (NICE, 2008b) and the Standards for Maternity Care developed by the relevant Royal Colleges in the UK (RCOG, 2008), provide guidance for improvement in both the safety and the experience of maternity care for the infant and the mother. These highlight the overarching need to have a strong midwifery workforce to support women and their partners during pregnancy, birth and early parenthood, deliver services which avoid unnecessary intervention, and ensure that those women who do, or may require intervention are directed at an early stage to specialist care.

One of the most important interventions prior to a child's birth which, on the basis of good evidence, has the potential to reduce inequalities in health, is smoking cessation.

Smoking cessation

Smoking during pregnancy has been shown to have detrimental effects on babies and mothers. A range of strategies have been attempted in order to help pregnant women reduce the number of cigarettes they smoke or stop smoking, with varying rates of success. A systematic review (Lumley et al., 2009) found a total of 72 controlled trials involving over 25,000 women mainly in high-income countries. The most effective intervention appeared to be providing incentives, which helped around 24% of women who received this intevention to quit. The smoking cessation interventions reduced the number of preterm births and of babies with low birthweight. Guidance on quitting smoking during pregnancy and following childbirth (NICE, 2010a) provides evidence-informed information on how to go about this.

This is one of the areas where qualitative research throws light on the contextual factors that can help to explain that mothers smoking in pregnancy isn't simply because of a lack of knowledge of the consequences. Stress – 'I smoke more if I've got bills coming in' – and creating space and time for themselves – 'just wait until I've finished this cigarette' – are among the reasons; this is in addition to the known addictive properties of tobacco, which cause some women to find it hard to give up, as described in Hilary Graham's (1993b) finely textured qualitative work on smoking.

In infancy

Breastfeeding is a key intervention for which the evidence base is strong (although stronger on benefits to children than on successful ways to close the gap between the better-off mothers and the less well off).

Breastfeeding

Breastfeeding is a key determinant of the nutrition, health, development and emotional well-being of infants, and of long-term health gains extending into adulthood, yet there are marked socioeconomic, ethnic and regional differences in starting to breastfeed, and then continuing. These differences can contribute to both initial and persistent inequalities in health. Babies who are not breastfed are many times more likely to acquire infections such as gastroenteritis in their first year (Horta et al., 2007). If all UK infants were exclusively breastfed, it is estimated that the number hospitalised each month with diarrhoea would be halved, and the number hospitalised with a respiratory infection would be cut by a quarter (Quigley et al., 2007).

Breastfeeding is associated with a number of benefits to children, and can be a source of pleasure to mothers (Thompson and Westreich, 1989). It is cheap (though not without additional costs for a good diet to the mother) and convenient and is associated with lower rates of infection and lower rates of sudden infant death.

Around two thirds of babies in the UK have some breastfeeding. Better-off mothers are more likely to breastfeed, and to breastfeed for longer. One well-designed randomised trial examined the effects of feeding the baby soon after birth and not restricting the timing of feeds after that. Women who fed their babies within two hours of birth and subsequently on demand continued to breastfeed for longer and had fewer problems than women who delayed the first feed for four hours and who fed on a fixed schedule (Salariya et al., 1978; Garcia et al., 1994). Garcia and her colleagues have also pointed out that this is an area where there is a gap between policies and practice. Maternity units with formal policies which encourage contact between mothers and babies, or breastfeeding soon after delivery, have been observed not to adhere to this in practice (Garforth and Garcia, 1989). Studies of the provision of free samples of artificial milk, while methodologically flawed, suggest, unsurprisingly, that this is associated with discontinuation of breastfeeding (Garcia et al., 1994).

A review from the NHS Centre for Reviews and Dissemination (CRD, 2000) suggests that small group informal discussions appear to be the most effective way to encourage breastfeeding, with educational leaflets largely ineffective, and a Cochrane review on skin to skin contact between mothers and babies at birth (Moore et al., 2007), also referred to in Chapter Seven, suggests that this simple cost-free intervention may well have good outcomes in the future as well as in the here and now. The review included 30 studies involving 1,925 mothers and their babies and showed that babies interacted more with their mothers, stayed warmer, and cried less if they had early skin-to-skin contact. They were also more likely to be breastfed, and to breastfeed for longer.

NICE (2011) found that most established peer and professional educational breastfeeding interventions were estimated to be cost-effective, even when the resulting health benefits were conservatively estimated. Indeed, if it is accepted that demonstrable health benefits in later life (for example, reduced risk of cardiovascular disease) are causally associated with breastfeeding, then virtually all breastfeeding schemes are cost-effective, and often extremely so.

Qualitative evidence provides a further dimension. One well-designed study concluded that women were keen to maintain ownership, control and responsibility for their own decision making about infant feeding and, not surprisingly, their core goal a contented baby. They viewed the goal for health professionals as the continuation of breastfeeding. These differences can give rise to dissatisfaction with communication, which is often seen as 'breastfeeding-centred' rather than 'woman-centred'. The authors suggest that verbal advice is insufficient, and that what women value is being shown how to feed their baby. Spending time with a caring midwife was highly valued (Hoddinott and Pill, 2000). This was reinforced by the findings of an intervention study using an action research model in a rural area of Scotland (Hoddinott et al., 2006). While acknowledging the problems of interpretation given that this was not an RCT, the intervention increased breastfeeding initiation and duration, and most effectively so for women giving birth and receiving postnatal care in a midwife-led community unit in the intervention area – something which has implications for the organisation of maternity care.

NICE makes recommendations to commissioners, mothers and others on the basis of the evidence. As well as the broad-brush principles, this includes very practical advice for mothers who may be returning to work, and need to know how to continue to breastfeed their baby. The box below gives one such example.

- Show all breastfeeding mothers how to hand-express breast milk.
- Advise mothers that expressed milk can be stored for:
  - up to five days in the main part of a fridge, at 4°C or lower
  - up to two weeks in the freezer compartment of a fridge
  - up to six months in a domestic freezer, at minus 18°C or lower.
- Advise mothers who wish to store expressed breast milk for less than five days that the fridge preserves its properties more effectively than freezing.
- Advise mothers who freeze their expressed breast milk to defrost it in the fridge and not to re-freeze it once thawed. Advise them never to use a microwave oven to warm or defrost breast milk.

For further details, see NICE (2011)

Pre-school children

For pre-school children, evidence supports the use of:

- affordable high-quality day care and education (Zoritch et al., 2000; Marmot, 2010);
- family and parenting support (Barlow et al., 2010).

Support and day care in the early years form an important component of thinking on reducing inequalities in health, but it is the 'high quality' element which is crucial. The first nursery school in England was started in 1914 by early years pioneers Margaret and Rachel McMillan – an 'open air' nursery which marked the beginnings of a movement that spread across the world, some of the ideas of which were underpinned by Margaret McMillan's *Education through the imagination* (McMillan, 1904). We know that education 'works'. The cohort studies show that both early education and parental support for education are strongly associated with overcoming early disadvantage. The Cochrane review of day care is summarised in the next box.

Day care for pre-school children

Day care increases children's IQ and has beneficial effects on behavioural development and school achievement. Long-term follow-up demonstrates increased employment, lower teenage pregnancy rates, higher socioeconomic status and decreased criminal behaviour. There are positive effects on mothers' education, employment and interaction with children. Effects on fathers have not been examined. Few studies look at a range of outcomes spanning the health, education and welfare domains. Most of the trials combined non-parental day care with some element of parent training or education (mostly targeted at mothers).

The authors caution that trials had other significant methodological weaknesses, pointing to the importance of improving on study design in this field. All the trials were carried out in the US (Zoritch et al., 2000).

Emotional and behavioural problems in children are common. A Cochrane review by Barlow et al. (2010) which is applicable to parents and carers of children up to three years eleven months, provides some support for the use of group-based parenting programmes to improve the emotional and behavioural adjustment of children in this age group, although there is insufficient evidence to reach firm conclusions regarding the role that such programmes might play in the primary prevention of such problems. There are also limited data available concerning the long-term effectiveness of these programmes.

Cost-effectiveness and early intervention

One piece of research evidence which made early use of cost-benefit data, and is referred to in the previous chapter, has had a significant effect and is described in brief in the next box.

Perry Pre-School Programme

A long-term study of the High/Scope Perry Pre-School Programme, launched in an impoverished Michigan community in the US, has provided influential evidence that high-quality pre-school education can exert a lasting, positive influence over children's lives. The programme randomly assigned more than 120 children aged three and four to a control group or an experimental group which was given good-quality pre-school for up to two years. The latter attended class for 2.5 hours a day for 30 weeks a year. Each family received a weekly home visit of 1.5 hours, and educational attainment and other aspects of the children's lives were monitored through to adulthood. By the age of 19, it was apparent that, compared with the control group, those who had attended pre-school were less likely to have needed special educational support, more likely to have completed their schooling and more likely to have found a job. Girls were less likely to have become pregnant (Berrueta-Clement et al., 1984).

At age 27, graduates of the High/Scope programme had:

- significantly higher monthly earnings (29% vs 7% earning $2,000 or more per month);
- a significantly higher percentage of home ownership (36% vs 13%);
- a significantly higher level of schooling completed (71% vs 54% completing 12th grade or higher);
- a significantly lower percentage receiving social services at some time in the last 10 years (59% vs 80%);
- significantly fewer arrests (7% vs 35% with five or more).

It has been calculated that for every $1 originally invested in the Perry Pre-School Programme, there has been a return to the taxpayer in reduced crime and in lower demand for special education, welfare and other public services of over $7 in real terms (Barnett, 1993). Performance was, in turn, associated with fewer arrests and better job prospects (Schweinhart and Weikart, 1993).

While the programme has not been without its critics (and responses to criticisms) there can be no doubt that the combination of long-term follow-up and the costing data had a galvanising effect on early childhood policy worldwide.

Evidence also comes from the follow-up of a randomised controlled study of directive home visiting support for socially disadvantaged mothers. The study found significant effects on maternal and child functioning, including ameliorating effects on child abuse and neglect, maternal welfare dependence, adult and child alcohol and drug misuse problems, and child antisocial behaviour and criminality (Olds et al., 1998, 1999; Eckenrode et al., 2010). This programme is now being rolled out as the Family Nurse Partnership (FNP) in the UK (see the next box). FNP is a licensed programme, developed in the US at the University of Colorado, where it is known as the Nurse Family Partnership (NFP). It is a preventive programme for young first-time mothers offering intensive and structured home visiting, delivered by family nurses from early pregnancy until the child is two. The programme aims to improve pregnancy outcomes, child health and development and parents' economic self-sufficiency. Methods are based on theories of human ecology, self-efficacy and attachment, with much of the work focused on building strong relationships between the client and family nurse to facilitate behaviour change and tackle the emotional problems that prevent some mothers and fathers caring well for their child.

It needs to be remembered that the UK already has a long history of health visitors seeing mothers at home, which may well mean less impressive results from an intervention originally designed and delivered in a country where there is no such service, and where outcomes for children are less positive than in the UK.

The Family Nurse Partnership (FNP)

FNP has been tested in England since 2007 and there are currently teams in 50 areas. The Department of Health (DH) is evaluating the programme with a three-year formative evaluation, and a large-scale research trial is due to report in due course.

The DH reports that the potential for early impacts and for cost savings look encouraging, with families valuing the programme less likely to smoke in pregnancy and more likely to breastfeed. In addition, at the end of the programme, they report that mothers were very positive about their parenting capability; they had significantly improved mastery, a form of self-esteem linked to positive behaviour change; clients were returning to education and employment, making regular use of effective birth control methods and spacing subsequent pregnancies; and the children appear to be developing in line with the population in general, which is very promising as this group usually fare much worse.

Department of Health (nd)

An intervention which has received rather less attention is the Community Mothers Programme (CMP) which grew out of the Early Childhood Development Programme designed in Bristol, UK, and which was piloted in the Republic of Ireland in 1988. In its current form, it is being delivered to nearly 1,200 parents each year in the Dublin area. CMP trains experienced mothers from the local community to visit families to provide childrearing support. It is focused on the child, but there is evidence that the community benefits, especially in relation to the sense of empowerment experienced by volunteers and parents, are more general. CMP operates mainly in disadvantaged neighbourhoods and is offered to parents – first timers and some second timers – of children from birth to 24 months. It aims to aid the development of parenting skills and enhance parents' confidence and self-esteem. It is an important aspect of the approach that community mothers should reflect the ethos of the community they intend to visit. This makes it less likely that mothers will feel that help, support and advice are being offered with any suggestion of condescension, or 'bossiness'. The wider motivation is to introduce solidarity to a community based on an exchange of knowledge and experience. There are indications that participation helps to increase feelings of self-worth among the volunteers, as they see the parents they are supporting gaining an understanding of child development. In the process, they gain status within their own community. A recent study also showed that volunteering in the programme contributed to lifelong learning (Molloy, 2007). At the same time, parents are encouraged to believe in their own capabilities and skills without becoming dependent on professionals. Community mothers are recruited, trained and supported by family development nurses. Each full-time family development nurse works with a team of 18–20 community mothers and supports 100–120 families at any one time. Family development nurses are in turn supported by a programme director who offers specialist support, education and management in the development, implementation and maintenance of the programme. The development of a programme in an area takes 18–24 months.

Community mothers visit parents once a month in their own homes armed with a set of strategies focusing on health care, nutrition and overall child development. They are given nominal expenses for each visit. They typically spend upwards of 13 hours each month on their visits to between five and fifteen families. The focus is a monthly family visit when parents – mothers and fathers alike – are encouraged to set themselves goals for the month ahead. Issues discussed at each session are tailored to the particular needs of the family. The approach supports the parents' own ideas and acknowledges that they will want to do what is best for their child. Additional help, such as breastfeeding support groups and parent and toddler groups, has evolved over the years. They are facilitated by community mothers and support an additional 600 parents each year.

The CMP has never attracted the same attention as some of the programmes from further afield, despite positive results. The most recent annual report (HSE and Molloy, 2011) describes positive outcomes for everything from immunisation to reading with the child.

In terms of research, in the 1990s CMP was subject to an RCT (Johnson et al., 1993) and found to have significant beneficial effects for mothers and children. Children in the programme scored better in terms of immunisation, language, education and cognitive development and nutrition, and their mothers scored better in terms of nutrition and self-esteem. At that time, the programme was only aimed at first-time parents during the first 12 months of the child's life; parents received a maximum of 12 visits, usually one a month lasting approximately one hour. Further evaluation was conducted seven years later when the children were aged eight (Johnson et al., 2000). A major finding was the persistence of parenting skills among the programme families. Children whose mothers were in the CMP were more likely to have better nutritional intake, to read books and to visit the library regularly. Mothers in the programme also had higher levels of self-esteem. They were more likely to oppose smacking, have strategies to help them and their children to deal with conflict, enjoy participating in their children's games, eat appropriate foods and express positive feelings about motherhood. The benefits of the CMP also extended to subsequent births: children were more likely to have completed their primary and MMR immunisation and to be breastfed. There were indications that just 12 contact hours in the first year of a child's life can make a difference.

An intervention not to be tried at home

In an article in the *Lancet*, entitled 'Mental contentment and physical growth', Widdowson (1951) described an experiment which could not be replicated, for reasons which will become obvious, but which underlines the importance of loving care (see the next box).

Food, care and understanding context

Near an industrial town in Germany in 1948 were two orphanages, each housing about 50 boys and girls aged 4 to 14. These children had only their official rations, which were barely adequate. The children were weighed and measured every fortnight for a year. During the second six months, one of the homes ('Vogelnest') was provided with unlimited additional bread, as well as jam and concentrated orange juice. The children at the other home ('Bienenhaus') continued with their normal rations.

During the first six months (when no extra food was supplied) children at Vogelnest gained more on average than the children in Bienenhaus. During the second six months, in spite of extra rations going to Vogelnest, the Bienenhaus children started to do much better.

The researchers investigated what else was going on. In 1948, Bienenhaus was in the charge of a Fräulein Schwarz, who was rather forbidding. Children and staff lived in fear of her reprimands, frequently delivered at mealtimes. At the time that food was increased at Vogelnest, she was transferred there, together with some favourite children whom she took with her. While they were at the first home, these children had gained more weight than the others, and on transfer to the second home, where the extra food was provided they put on weight very rapidly. Widdowson concluded, 'This kind of experiment is difficult to 'repeat' or 'confirm', but there is no doubt that even the most perfectly planned nutritional investigation may be ruined by psychological factors over which the investigator may have no control. Those about to embark on feeding experiments would do well to remember: 'Better a dinner of herbs where love is served than a stalled ox and hatred therewith' (Widdowson, 1951: 318).

What is as important as the later outcomes are the good childhood experiences in the here and now, and the enjoyment which children gain from these early encounters. Childhood is not just a period of training for being a grown-up.

Key messages

General
* Delivering good outcomes for children is a tall order when we know that modest interventions usually have modest effects. This makes careful selection of the interventions most likely to be beneficial all the more necessary.
* If it is impossible to find good evidence, or the systematic reviews encourage taking interventions from elsewhere a step further, partnerships can enable practitioners and researchers to carry out a really robust evaluation. This means that even if it doesn't have the expected results, the work will contribute to the knowledge base of what works.

Day care and early education
* The quality and the content of pre-school provision matters.
* Poor day care may do more harm than good.

- Pre-school education can improve longer-term outcomes for disadvantaged children.
- Staff should be well-trained in child development, and well supported to encourage minimal turnover.

Social support
- Social and emotional support can make a difference. If an intervention or service which does this is being considered, the systematic reviews on what seems to make the greatest difference should be used.
- We need to know more about what kinds of parenting education and support work, and we will only know this with well-designed and well-evaluated interventions. As well as published trials and reviews, others are in progress.

Breastfeeding
- Breastfeeding is associated with better outcomes for babies.
- Giving women leaflets is of little value.
- Hospitals whose policies support breastfeeding need to ensure that their practices are in line with their policies.

Smoking reduction or cessation
In addition to the positive effects of legislative changes:
- Nicotine replacement therapy is effective.
- Generic self-help materials are no better than brief advice but more effective than doing nothing. Personalised materials are more effective than standard materials.
- Brief advice from doctors and nurses increases the quit rate and more intensive advice is slightly more effective.
- Brief cognitive behavioural interventions, with support, appear to be helpful in reducing passive smoking in households where the mother smokes.
- The use of incentives in smoking cessation appears to be promising.

FOUR

What works in childhood and adolescence?

Much research and intervention effort over the last decade or so has focused on infancy and early childhood. While this is important, it is also important not to let messages about the plasticity of the brain in infancy feed into a perception that the die is cast by the time a child hits primary school. Recent work on stroke in much older people, for instance, has demonstrated that the capacity for recovery is much greater than used to be thought, and greater throughout life.

There are many ways in which inequalities in health and their causes and consequences can be addressed throughout childhood and adolescence. We know that education has great potential to level the playing field overall. But it is both a powerful means of combating inequalities, and a field where inequalities persist. Problems of bullying, obesity, smoking and substance abuse, emotional ill health and teenage pregnancy are all areas with a growing body of research designed to inform policy and practice.

The evidence, as Jessop (2006) has suggested, is frustrating. Some of the best evaluated programmes have modest effects, but at a population level, these modest effects can make a real difference. Other studies may show dramatic effects, but be constructed on the basis of small numbers, or use methods which may tell us things we need to know, but not the crucial thing – does this do more good than harm?

What are the problems?

Chapter One describes the fall in mortality in childhood and adolescence. But at the same time, there has been an increase in some chronic health problems which cannot be explained simply by improved diagnosis. Both asthma and diabetes, for instance, are on the increase. For most children and adolescents, the periods after infancy and before adulthood are a time when health inequalities are not as stark (West, 1997; Spencer, 2006). However, given that the effects of inequalities in health and in life are cumulative, developing right across the life course, this is a time when there is potential for setting in place the building blocks for good health. Adolescence is a time of experimentation, and as Viner and Barker (2005) point out, risk behaviours, including binge drinking, criminal activity and using illegal drugs, may contribute to the development of both health and social inequalities during the transition from adolescence to adulthood (West, 1997). They also point out that, since the adolescent population is more ethnically diverse than older groups, health inequalities linked with ethnicity disproportionately affect young people.

What are some of the solutions?

As Chapter Two describes, the cohort studies provide an important source of knowledge on the ways in which some children with a poor start to life nevertheless achieve good outcomes. There is a good deal to be learned from these studies about the promotion of resilience. A key element in achieving this is a good educational start. There is a growing number of well-evaluated intervention studies in school and community settings, and over the next few years the accumulated evidence from these is likely to be helpful in better understanding the most effective and cost-effective interventions, and in considering the ways in which these might be used in different contexts.

One of the problems of looking for evidence to support interventions is that it may well feed into a deficit model – 'this is broken – how do we fix it?' Most problems do not come along in ones, and interventions at the community or school level are more difficult to evaluate well. Education is itself a complex intervention, and one which, as the cohort studies demonstrate, has (relatively speaking) a good, if far from perfect track record in addressing inequality. The ability of children and young people to counter at least some of the disadvantages they are exposed to is further reason why any intervention should be informed by listening to children and young people themselves to enable policy and practice to go with the grain of those it is designed to support.

Education

Universal education, as every development agency knows, is the single intervention that can make the greatest difference to a child's life and to the future of both the child and the nation. The link between education and health is well known. The period from the start of schooling until school leaving age is one of huge potential, as set out in the Marmot (2010) report, and education is one of the interventions capable of sustaining achievement at both the individual and the population level. Findings from the Centre for Research on the Wider Benefits of Learning show that there are returns to education in terms of self-reported health, lower mortality rates and lower incidence of depression and obesity, and in health-related behaviours such as diet, exercise, smoking, and take-up of preventive health care measures (Gutman et al., 2010). Quick and Wilkinson (1991) point out that the Chancellor of the Exchequer has a greater effect on health than the Secretary of State for Health. If that is so at a national and (in terms of global finance) increasingly at a supra-national level, as well as at an individual and community level, it is likely that in terms of long-term health prospects, gifted school teachers make an outstanding difference (Gutman and Feinstein, 2008).

But while education is a powerful tool for achieving other benefits, seeing school as simply one more way to bring about change across the life course gives a focus on becoming an adult (which is important, but not all-important). Also important is being a child and enjoying it. In 2011, the *Guardian* newspaper asked children to dream up their perfect school and compiled some of their replies into a Children's Manifesto. Some of the creative and heartwarming ideas they came up with are summarised in the next box.

Life is not only the absence of ills ...

- **Calm** music instead of bells.
- **Comfortable** with big enough chairs, small enough chairs, and slippers.
- **Expert**: In the classroom we should have Stephen Hawking to teach us science. I would like Gordon Ramsay to cook our lunch, but he would have to promise to zip his mouth.
- **Flexible**: If we're doing something that needs a lot of thinking, there should be enough time to finish.
- **Friendly**, with kind teachers who speak softly and don't shout.
- **Listening**: Children should be listened to because they sometimes have better ideas than adults. That is because the children's brains are new and not old.
- **Inclusive**: It's unfair that only the people who are good at writing stories have their stories displayed in the school hall. I think everyone should have their work displayed. That way no one feels left out.
- **International**: At lunchtime a buffet with Namibian, Chinese, Indian and French food would be served on flower-shaped plates and we would listen to music from that country as we ate.
- **Outside**: Fortnightly school trips (without worksheets), animals to look after like chickens, sheep and horses, and greenhouses to grow fruit and vegetables to eat at school and sell to raise funds.
- **Technological**: There should be digital recorders available for lessons, so if you go to the toilet, when you come back you can catch up on what you have missed.

What the perfect school would have

- **No homework** (all the work would be finished at school).
- **Pets**: 'Bring dogs to school in case we need a friend'.
- **Fewer tests** (but not no tests at all).

Birkett (2011)

What helps?

Even in countries with universal education, access can be problematic, with children from the most disadvantaged backgrounds being those most likely to be truanting or excluded from school for misbehaviour, or placed in the bottom sets (Dunne et al., 2007; Dyson and Gallannaugh, 2008; DCSF, 2009). Poor educational attainment is related to health directly (with more smoking, for instance, among those who do less well) and later on through the kinds of jobs which people do (Hammond and Feinstein, 2006).

While schools can be successful in attempts to promote health directly, the evidence from studies on health education is not very strong and some of the most robust studies come from other countries and contexts, with no guarantee that their findings are transferable (Lister-Sharp et al., 1999; Warwick et al., 2009). Stewart-Brown (2006) reports even more limited effects from programmes targeting substance misuse and suicide. Many evaluations focus on relatively short-term impacts, in terms of changes in attitudes and health-related behaviours during and immediately after participation in programmes. It is less clear whether the impacts of programmes are sustained in the long term and whether, therefore, they have impacts on adult health.

Currently, approaches to complex interventions and whole-school approaches look likely to change the way we look at these problems (Bonell et al., 2007; Bond and Butler, 2009). Butler et al. (2010) also argue for the need to move beyond conventional dissemination strategies to a focus on active partnerships between developers and users of school-based intervention research, and they offer a conceptual tool for planning dissemination. Risk behaviours such as smoking, drinking and drug use, as well as sexual risk and violence, as Viner and Barker (2005) make clear, often come together. Interventions which build on this, rather than focus on each risk separately are more likely to be helpful.

If education is to 'work' at its best, it is important to recognise that some of the elements which are problematic are both those which children themselves define as problematic such as bullying, and those which the cohort studies have demonstrated to be problematic, such as a lack of parental engagement in a child's education, and truanting and exclusion.

Tackling bullying

Bullying is a type of aggressive behaviour (although it does not always involve violence), and is included here as it has been consistently identified by children as important to them, although it has frequently been swept under the carpet or redefined as 'teasing' or 'a bit of fun'. Bullying is the single biggest problem presented by children phoning ChildLine. In 2007/08, 32,562 children and young people spoke to them about bullying as their main problem, representing 18 per cent of all calls answered (ChildLine, 2008).

Bullying is not restricted to school but it frequently has its origins there. This kind of behaviour can have serious physical and mental health consequences for both bullies and bullied. Being bullied can have a long-term impact and contribute to poor mental health, trouble with personal relationships and unemployment risk in adulthood (Hugh-Jones and Smith, 1999). Rothon et al. (2011), drawing on an East London study found that being bullied had a strong impact on adolescents' chances of achieving the national academic benchmark for their age. One possible mechanism they suggest is that according to Smith et al. (2004), bullied children are more likely to play truant or be absent from school for other reasons. Rothon and her colleagues showed that support from friends and family alone was not able to mitigate against the strong negative effect that bullying had on mental health among the secondary school pupils they studied in East London.

Figure 4.1: 'Stop bullying now' (drawing by primary school pupil, Glasgow)

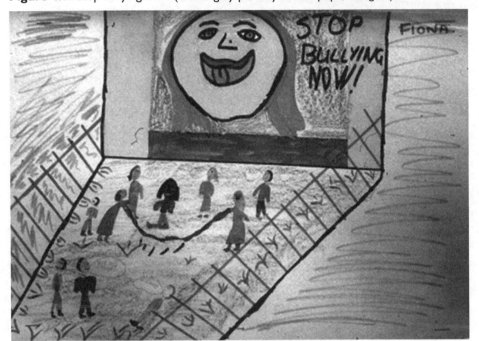

A systematic review (Farrington and Ttofi, 2010) identified 89 studies which were sufficiently robustly designed to meet their eligibility criteria. The authors found that some elements of school-based anti-bullying programmes seem to be effective, reducing bullying by 20–23% and victimisation by 17–20%. Not everything worked, and work with peers was significantly associated with an increase in victimisation. The duration and intensity of the programme, parent training/meetings, and disciplinary methods seem to have been associated with a good effect. The review found that bullied children often don't communicate to anyone what is happening to them. Programmes in Norway seem to work best, which the authors suggest may be due to the longer tradition of anti-bullying programmes and evaluations there.

A review of cyber bullying (Mishna et al., 2009) was not quite so promising in its assessment of the evidence. The authors found that while participation in internet safety interventions is associated with an increase in internet safety knowledge, it does not change risky online behaviour. Other kinds of evaluations present more promising findings, although these tend to be based on methods which may tell a good narrative (unlike most systematic reviews), often using self-report or rating scales. These too are an important source of data, and should not be dismissed, but nor should they be confused with sound evidence.

Parental support for, or involvement in, education

Parental support for, and involvement in, education is one of the most important factors in improving outcomes for children who have had a poor start in life. Children fortunate enough to have this help are much more likely to do well at school (Douglas, 1986). In due course, such children as adults are more likely to be enthusiastic about their own children's education (Wadsworth, 1991). Many of the parents who find it difficult to take an interest in or be involved in their child's education may not themselves have had positive experiences of school. In looking at what helps, a systematic review has examined approaches to parental involvement for improving the academic performance of elementary school age children (Nye et al., 2006).

The types of parent involvement in the studies in the review included:

- collaborative reading
- maths games
- reading games
- education and training in doing maths, science or other learning activities with their children
- rewards and incentives provided by the parents for their children's performance in school.

The authors found that parental involvement, defined as parents engaging their children in activities to enhance academic performance, has a significant positive effect on children's overall academic achievement. The academic area most positively affected was reading, and the types of parent involvement which had the greatest impact were rewards and incentives provided by parents to their children outside the school day for performance in school, and education and training provided to parents. The reported effect was large enough to have practical implications for parents, family involvement practitioners and policy makers. Even when parents participated in academic enrichment activities with their children outside of school for an average of less than 12 weeks, children demonstrated an equivalent of four to five months' improvement in reading or maths performance.

Tutoring

Tutoring is a method sometimes used by middle-class parents to support their child's education, or to support entry to competitive private schools. They clearly believe that it has an effect, and it may do. Less is known about tutoring in other contexts. Systematic reviews of volunteer tutoring in elementary and middle schools by Ritter et al. (2006, 2009) found that compared to non-tutored peers, children with volunteer tutors seemed to do better on letters, words and writing assessments and oral skills, but very little is known about the effectiveness of volunteer tutoring for maths outcomes. Any roll-out of tutoring could be tied in with a trial. However, effectiveness trials alone are unlikely to be useful without studies of process issues such as who organises tutoring in the school, whether the tutors are safe, available and reliable, and when they provide the tutoring. Involving children, teachers, classroom assistants and parents in designing the form if not the content of tutoring schemes and then trialling it makes sense.

Figure 4.2: 'Don't leave us out'

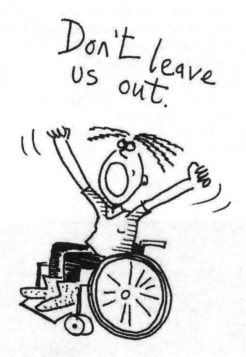

© Angela Martin

Adapted from Don't leave us out: Involving disabled children and young people with communication impairments by Jenny Morris, published in 1998 by the Joseph Rowntree Foundation. Reproduced by permission of the Joseph Rowntree Foundation and Angela Martin.

Disabled children and their families

Disabled children may have additional needs, but on the whole they want to learn, play, have friends, and get out and about in much the same way as other children and young people. Their parents tend to want the same, and the chance to parent without also becoming their child's key worker, co-ordinating the appointments and undertaking the large amount of form filling that services for disabled children tend to require. Difficulties in using public transport, as well as the cost, make access to positive activities challenging for disabled children and young people, and this has knock-on effects for families and parental employment (Sloper, 1999). There is, however, work in progress with the aim of addressing this (Andrews, 2009).

> 'It doesn't matter how good things are, if you can't get there in the first place, what's the point?' (Young person) (Beresford and Clarke, 2010)

When I saw this car (Figure 4.3) on a disabled parking space in central London, I liked to think that it was full of young people, some disabled, some not, ready for a good night out.

When Beresford et al. (1996) wrote their *What works for families with a disabled child*, they pointed out that the relative lack of direct research with disabled children themselves would have made *What works for disabled children* (rather than for their families) problematic as a title. Since then, there has been some progress, but as The Centre for Excellence and Outcomes (C4EO) points out, we still know far too little about the views of young disabled children, and have a lack of really robust research evidence on interventions.

Disabling attitudes and unequal access to education, health care and other services, are key problems. Disability and poverty are inter-linked, as the next box demonstrates.

Figure 4.3: Disabled car

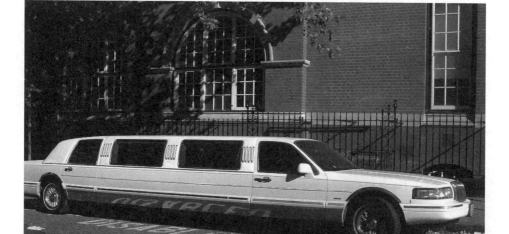

Reproduced with permission from BMJ Publishing Group; from Roberts, H. 'Disabled stretch limo', *Journal of Epidemiology and Community Health*, 2008, 62:565, doi:10.1136/jech.2007.07193.

> • A report from Contact a Family (Bennett, 2010) repeated a survey of families with a disabled child first carried out in 2008. They found that almost a quarter are going without heating (23%) up from 16% in 2008.
> • One in seven (14%) are going without food, down from 16% in 2008.
> • More than half (51%) have borrowed money from family or friends to keep financially afloat or pay for essentials such as food and heating, up from 42% in 2008.
> • Minority ethnic families with a disabled child are more likely to be living in difficult circumstances, with lower levels of both support and benefit (Chamba et al., 1999).

Given differing definitions of disability, different age groups and with differing levels of confidence, it is hard to give a clear metric for disability in general (Blackburn et al., 2007; Read et al., 2010). Mooney et al. (2008) point out that planning and improving services require good data, and their best estimate, on the basis of research, is that between 3 and 5.4% of children under 18 years are disabled.

What helps?

The work of the Social Policy Research Unit (SPRU) at the University of York, among others, has been groundbreaking in addressing the things that matter to disabled children and their families. They have developed and sustained studies on key workers, and looked at some of the important day-to-day issues faced by all families, but often more starkly by families where there is a disabled child, such as the child's (and hence the parent's) sleep. They (Beresford and Clarke, 2010), and Tony Newman (Newman, 2010; Newman et al., 2010) from Barnardo's have fed in extensively to the evidence reviews for C4EO.

Among the key findings of the reviews are that:

• families of young disabled children who have a consistent key worker will usually experience better relationships with services, quicker access to benefits, and reduced stress; and that
• high-quality pre-school education can reduce the need for special education at primary school, especially for the most disadvantaged children.

What helps in terms of inclusion seems to be:

• skilled and knowledgeable practitioners;
• all staff working proactively to support and facilitate inclusion;
• types of activities that support and facilitate inclusion;
• the provision of adequate information about the service;
• support tailored to the needs of disabled users;
• support to the service from health professionals;
• continuity of staff and venue.

Beresford and Clarke (2010) suggest that things are improving in this direction, but there is more to be done.

It is frequently difficult to work out from published sources how one might even start to think about an intervention. A refreshingly detailed example of local practice provided as an example of good practice by C4EO is summarised in the next box.

Hull Aiming High Cycling Scheme

East Park, in Hull, is 140 acres of green space offering an animal and education centre, youth zone and water play areas. There are mobility scooters available for people who have problems getting around. The park has a Sustrans route and an inner road for cycling. The cycling scheme has created opportunities for disabled children and young people to be able to cycle with their mum, dad, brother, sister, friends and carers. The children and young people who access the scheme have a wide range of disabilities including learning disabilities, physical disabilities, autism and complex health needs. All the special schools in Hull have become members of the scheme and use cycling as part of their curriculum and activity programme.

The plan for the cycling scheme was endorsed by the Aiming High Board and the Hull Children's Trust Board, and also agreed through the Hull Parents Forum, a group of parents and carers of disabled children who for the first time jointly commissioned, with the local authority and health service, all of the short-break programmes under the scheme. Four young people joined representatives from Hull City Council and others on a Steering Group.

Two part-time city council administration staff were relocated to the park, allowing rangers more time to be involved in the cycling scheme. The Youth Service offered to fund a full-time worker. The intention of the scheme was always to embed it within the park's own facilities and to ensure that the scheme was sustainable once the project had been completed. The website describing the scheme in more detail includes such crucial details as costings, service level agreements with repairers, pictures of the cycles and details of suppliers.

www.c4eo.org.uk/themes/disabledchildren/vlpdetails.aspx?lpeid=318

Adolescence

The great majority of adolescents are not problem people with problem lives, but face the same difficulties as everyone else, while still serving an apprenticeship in how to deal with those difficulties. The routine and casual vilification of young people in the press and elsewhere may be one of the greatest problems many of them face. That said, in addressing inequalities in health, it would be reckless to take no account of, for instance, Boreham and Blenkinsop's (2004) report that:

- a third of 15-year-olds in England take illegal drugs and about a quarter use them monthly or more;
- among the 40% of 15-year-olds who drink alcohol, average weekly consumption is over 10 units;
- a quarter of 15-year-old girls smoke.

Teenage pregnancy

Pregnancy is not in itself a problem behaviour, but the circumstances of pregnancy may have consequences for the health and wider life chances of both the mother and the child. Lawlor and Shaw (2004) point out that we should be wary of moral panics and of claims that the rate of teenage pregnancy in Britain is 'high' and increasing. As a result of earlier sexual activity, the 'at-risk' population has risen sharply, but birth rates have not. This suggests that contrary to popular opinion, teenagers are reasonably competent at preventing unwanted pregnancies (Wellings and Kane, 1999). Lisa Arai (2009) has written compellingly on teenage pregnancy as the making and unmaking of a problem and the extent to which there is a focus on the problems of early motherhood, and little on the benefits or pleasures. That said, these pleasures and joys are likely to be reduced when those who become parents early or very early are more likely to be young people who:

- are living in deprived areas;
- do not attend school;
- are looked after by, or leaving local authority care services;
- are homeless.

But given that by no means all teenage pregnancies are unintended, unwanted or unplanned, supporting teenage mothers and their children is at least as important as preventing unwanted pregnancies. Many young mothers do well (Phoenix, 1990), including some young mothers leaving care. However, teenage pregnancy is often associated with poor health and social outcomes for both the mother and child. Young mothers are more likely to suffer postnatal depression and less likely to complete their education. Children born to teenage parents are less likely to be breastfed, more likely to live in poverty and more likely to become teenage parents themselves (Botting et al., 1998).

While 'sex education' has sometimes been seen as the key, there is stronger evidence that good basic education is protective, providing as it does a route into different life choices for young women (Arblaster et al., 1997). Those who have more years of education are less likely to become pregnant, as they have a range of options.

What may not help

> ### Not everything we want to be effective shows an effect in the desired direction
>
> A study to evaluate the effectiveness of youth development in reducing teenage pregnancy, substance use and other outcomes reported less than positive results. In a prospective matched comparison study at 54 youth service sites in England, young people were offered an intensive, multi-component youth development programme including sex and drugs education (Young People's Development Programme – YPDP) versus standard youth provision. The 2,724 young people in the programme, aged 13–15 years at baseline, were deemed by professionals to be at risk of teenage pregnancy, substance misuse or school exclusion, or to be vulnerable in other ways. Unexpectedly, the researchers' analysis suggested that participation in the YPDP was associated with higher rates of some harmful or potentially harmful outcomes than occurred at comparison sites. Among young women, YPDP participants more commonly reported teenage pregnancies, early heterosexual sex and the expectation of becoming a teenage parent, as well as temporary exclusion from school and truancy. The authors conclude that: 'No evidence was found that the intervention was effective in delaying heterosexual experience or reducing pregnancies, drunkenness, or cannabis use. Some results suggested an adverse effect. Although methodological limitations may at least partly explain these findings, any further implementation of such interventions in the UK should be only within randomised trials' (Wiggins et al., 2009).

Where we need to know more

Given that the children of teenage parents can have poor outcomes, and young parents themselves have a tough job, Barlow et al. (2011) carried out a systematic review to examine whether individual and group-based parenting programmes improve psychosocial outcomes for teenage parents and their children. A range of interventions are being used to promote the well-being of teenage parents and their children. Parenting programmes have been found to be effective in improving psychosocial health in parents more generally (including reducing anxiety and depression, and improving self-esteem), alongside a range of developmental outcomes for children. This review investigated the impact of parenting programmes aimed specifically at teenage parents. Results from four meta-analyses suggest that parenting programmes may be effective in improving parent responsiveness to the child, and parent–child interaction. Infant responsiveness to the mother also showed improvement at follow-up. Other analyses they carried out were inconclusive, suggesting that more research is needed.

Young smokers

Smoking has been identified as a core reason for the gap in life expectancy between rich and poor. Moreover, children who smoke become addicted to nicotine very quickly. They also tend to continue the habit into adulthood. Around two thirds of people who have smoked took up the habit before the age of 18 (Information Centre, 2006). Children and young people usually get cigarettes from friends, family and shops, especially small corner shops. However, they also buy from adults who sell them from home and from others involved in organised criminal activities.

Both European and North American studies have shown that parental opposition to smoking and setting clear standards about smoking are more important predictors of teenagers' intentions to smoke than parental smoking behaviour. This suggests that even if a parent is unable to give up smoking in order to set a good example, banning smoking at home may reduce teenage take-up (Aaro et al., 1981; Eiser et al., 1989; Mermelstein et al., 1999; Wakefield et al., 2000).

What works?

The National Institute for Health and Clinical Excellence (NICE) (2008a) and other guidance developed on the basis of research recommend sustained mass-media campaigns to prevent young people from taking up smoking. Campaigns should be developed with a range of partners, including national, regional and local government and non-governmental organisations, the National Health Service (NHS), children and young people, media professionals, public relations agencies and local anti-tobacco activists. The tobacco industry is not recommended as a partner in either development or delivery.

Local authorities are required to enforce legislation to prevent under-age tobacco sales under the Children and Young Persons (Protection from Tobacco) Act 1991. Making illegal tobacco sales a higher priority through increasing inspection and enforcement activities is likely to be effective if sustained, although recent austerity measures may make these activities less, not more likely.

Mass-media campaigns are usually run nationally by the Department of Health. However, it is likely that additional resources will be needed to deliver campaigns aimed at children and young people. The exact costs involved will depend on the aims and objectives of the activities delivered nationally, regionally and locally.

Mental health and substance abuse

Young people are frequently seen as more threatening than threatened, despite the evidence that they are more frequently the victims than the perpetrators of violent and other crime and the trauma of being a victim of crime can have damaging effects on mental health. Mental health is more profoundly affected by socioeconomic factors than many other dimensions of health (Carr–Hill et al., 1994). Up to 20% of all children and teenagers are maladjusted or distressed, although Goodman (1997) suggests that the medicalisation of distress is unhelpful. Buchanan and Ritchie (2004) suggest interventions with troubled young people, including programmes based on cognitive behavioural principles.

Among the guidance on what works in relation to mental health and associated problems are:

Parent-training/education programmes in the management of children with conduct disorders. NICE technology appraisal 102 (2006). Available from www.nice.org.uk/TA102.

Depression in children and young people: identification and management in primary, community and secondary care. NICE clinical guideline 28 (2005). Available from www.nice.org.uk/CG028.

Community-based interventions to reduce substance misuse among vulnerable and disadvantaged children and young people. NICE public health guidance 4 (2007). Available from www.nice.org.uk/PHI004.

Interventions in schools to prevent and reduce alcohol use among children and young people. NICE public health guidance 7 (2007). Available from www.nice.org.uk/PH007.

Promoting children's social and emotional wellbeing in primary education, NICE public health guidance 12 (2008) www.nice.org.uk/PH12.

Tackling obesity in children and young people

There is general guidance on maternal and child health nutrition from NICE on the prevention, identification, assessment and management of overweight and obesity in adults and children (NICE, 2006b, 2011). Almost 10% of children in reception classes (aged four–five) and 18.7% of children aged 10–11 are classified as obese (NCMP, 2009/2010).

Childhood overweight varies by ethnicity, socioeconomic circumstances, gender, age and population (Butland et al., 2007). Children in disadvantaged circumstances are more likely to be overweight or obese than their more advantaged peers and although trends in childhood obesity seem to be levelling off, socioeconomic differentials in childhood obesity rates may be widening. This may be because better-off families have been more likely, or more able to take on board messages promoting healthy patterns of diet and physical activity, more likely to access services which support behaviour change, or less likely to live in an obesogenic environment (Marmot et al., 2010). The effect of low income renders it meaningless to consider diet a matter solely of choice (Cole-Hamilton and Lang, 1986).

So far, evidence syntheses for the prevention or treatment of childhood overweight (Brown and Summerbell, 2009; Oude et al., 2009; SIGN, 2010; Whitlock et al., 2010;) have found insufficient evidence to recommend one programme over another, although principles of effective interventions have been established. These include addressing both diet and physical activity, behaviour change, involvement of family and a positive emphasis on managing a healthy lifestyle for the whole family. A recent mapping review of schemes to promote healthy weight among obese and overweight children in England found over 300 schemes with both practice and evaluation extremely variable (Aicken et al., 2010). While there are now tools for evaluation guidance on the National Obesity Observatory website,[1] these have come at a time when austerity funding is unlikely to make evaluation of projects at a local level a priority.

This chapter covers a long period in children's lives in a relatively short space by selecting only some of the areas where inequalities in health can be seen and may be remedied. Some of the issues here also apply to the children and young people in the next chapter.

What may not help

Pretty well nothing works in all circumstances all of the time, but the things that we should be wary of, or redesign in the light of some of the research evidence, do not always get quite as much coverage as the aspects of a service which do work. Practitioners are increasingly told what to add to their 'to do' lists without being told what might be taken off. The example in the next box suggests where disinvestment – or perhaps, better theorising, planning and implementation – might be considered.

Mentoring to prevent antisocial behaviour in childhood

Antisocial behaviour in childhood and adolescence is a problem for young people and their families, for health and welfare professionals planning multi-disciplinary services and for general practitioners approached by fraught parents (Webster Stratton, 1990; Scott et al., 2001). Antisocial behaviour in young people is also a problem for the police, for communities and for politicians. Behaviour problems in childhood can presage more serious problems in later life (Scott, 1998). This makes finding a solution a political as well as a therapeutic imperative – a potent driver to 'do something'.

One approach is through mentoring schemes. In a typical non-directive mentoring programme (which is the most common and promoted form of mentoring) a mentor will be a volunteer who provides support or guidance to someone younger or less experienced. The mentor aims to offer support, understanding, experience and advice. Mentoring is non-invasive and medication free. It is easy to see why it might work, and why it is attractive to politicians and policy makers. There is indeed robust research that indicates benefits from mentoring for some young people, for some programmes, in some circumstances, in relation to some outcomes (DuBois et al., 2002). There are also good descriptive evaluations which suggest

---

[1] www.noo.org.uk/core/eval_guidance

that those young people who stay on in programmes are inclined to report favourably on the experience (St James-Roberts and Samlal Singh, 2001; Tarling et al., 2001).

Where improvements have been reported, critical examination suggests flaws that weaken the conclusions. Mentoring programmes for vulnerable young people may have a negative impact, and adverse effects associated with mentor–mentee relationship breakdowns have been reported (Grossman and Rhodes, 2002). Worryingly, a 10-year follow-up study of one well-designed scheme unexpectedly found that a sub-group of mentored young people, some of whom had previously been arrested for minor offences, were more likely to be arrested after the project than those not mentored (O'Donnell and Lydgate, 1979). On the basis of findings such as these, and on the evidence available at the time, it was concluded that non-directive mentoring programmes delivered by volunteers cannot be recommended as an effective intervention for young people at risk for, or already involved in antisocial behaviour or criminal activities.

This does not mean that mentoring does not work. There are many different kinds of mentoring and some show better evidence of effect than others. Our current state of knowledge on the effectiveness of mentoring is similar to that of a new drug that shows promise, but remains in need of further research and development. There is no equivalent of NICE or Food and Drug Administration (FDA) for mentoring. If there were, no more than a handful of programmes might have realistic hopes of qualifying. And even then, it would have to be acknowledged that a full understanding of the safeguards needed to ensure that young people are not harmed by participation is lacking. For some of the most vulnerable young people, mentoring programmes as currently implemented may become one more intervention that fails to deliver on its promises.

Roberts et al. (2004b)

Key messages
- A good general education is strongly associated with health right across the life course, better skills, better employment prospects, and a lower likelihood of substance abuse and unintended teenage conceptions.
- Systematic review evidence suggests that there may well be effective interventions to tackle bullying (a high priority for children), to involve parents in schooling (which is associated with children with a poor start in life doing well), and to maintain discipline in the classroom.
- For young people who parent early or very early, education remains a key for both themselves and their children.
- The evidence base for effective interventions for disabled children and their families is growing. Some interventions, such as the cycling scheme in Hull, are also fun, and respond to the often expressed wish of disabled children and their families to be part of the crowd.

- There have been a number of attempts to address risky behaviours in young adulthood. These behaviours tend to be unresponsive to 'magic bullet' approaches, but interventions involving whole-school approaches look promising.

- Not every well-meaning intervention works, even if it looks as if it should. It is important to understand that most interventions have the capacity to do harm as well as good – even those that work for some people some of the time. That is what makes the evidence from trials particularly compelling. They do (or should) include drop-outs and those who don't take up the intervention, rather than simply interviewing and gaining self-reports on those who stay the course. It is always important to include responses from the children and adolescents involved in the evidence for deciding what to do and what not to do,. The wearer knows best where the shoe pinches.

FIVE

What works in keeping children safe?

Unintentional injury is an important cause of child death in the UK, with a steeper social class gradient for deaths than for any other cause of death in childhood and young adulthood. Despite the 'Keeping children safe' title of this chapter, child protection from intentional injury is only briefly referred to here, given that this important topic is well covered by an extensive literature, and data on the nature of inequalities in relation to child abuse are less clear.

Unlike child abuse, the dangers to children from accidental injury have seized the attention of neither the public nor the media. No director of children's services has been on the front of a tabloid or fired because the roads, the social housing stock or the lack of safe play areas on their patch represent a threat to children's lives and health. Unintentional injury is an area where relatively ineffective interventions, including exhortation and educational pamphlets, continue to be used, in spite of evidence of more effective ways of keeping children safe.

- A child from the lowest social class is 16 times more likely to die in a house fire than a child from a well-off home.
- Accidents are a major cause of death in childhood after the age of one in the UK.
- Child accidents are a cause of considerable morbidity in children and anxiety in adults.
- Accidents to under-fives are more likely to take place in the home, where they spend the majority of their time.
- Over-fives are more likely to have an accident in the external environment.
- The gap between the least and the most well off for accidental injury is not reducing, despite a reduction in accidental deaths overall.
- The reduction in road traffic injury and death to children is likely to have been bought at the expense of their life in the outdoors and their freedom to roam.

Background

The majority of children in Britain grow up in safe and loving families. But a number of children live all or some of their lives with danger (Lloyd et al., 1997). This can include hostile and unsafe urban environments, physical, emotional or sexual abuse or neglect, harassment, bullying or domestic violence. While considerable effort is put into addressing child protection in the private domain of the home and the family, in the public domain, a determined effort to address the issues which might prevent accidental injury has not occurred to anything like the same degree. Injury, however caused, is an important source of preventable harm.

There is probably no area of child health with as much ready potential to narrow inequalities as unintentional injury in the home and on the roads. There can also be few areas which attract such strong feelings from drivers reluctant to sacrifice speed or convenience, and from elements in the road lobby who resist a range of traffic calming measures as either unnecessary or as no more than a device for hidden taxation. An entire chapter is devoted to injury because this is the area of child health with the greatest differences between poor and rich children. The steep social gradient in child accidents was highlighted over thirty years ago in the Black report, and the inequalities they signalled were set out as important issues for investigation and action (Working Group on Inequalities in Health, 1980).

The terms 'unintentional injury' and 'accident' are both used in this chapter. Injury follows some, but not all accidents. The same event – a child sticking a knitting needle into an electric socket for instance – may have very different outcomes ranging from death to no injury at all. We need to know more about why some housing types, some roads, some communities and some schools are apparently more accident-prone than others. This involves collecting data on near-accidents and averted accidents as well as on the accidents which actually happen. Just as anaesthetists and those responsible for planes collect and analyse data on near-misses, more data, both quantitative and qualitative, is needed on dangerous places and events. Meanwhile, we need to use what is already known more effectively.

A fevered debate in the *British Medical Journal* followed a decision to ban the term 'accident', except in exceptional circumstances, and replace it with terms relating to the resulting injury (Davis and Pless, 2001). The correspondence which followed, both for and against the decision, included communications from epidemiologists, philosophers, social scientists and historians as well as physicians. One correspondent objecting to banning the term 'accident' pointed out that: 'At the level of population, most injuries are indeed predictable and preventable. At the individual level, in the "real world" where injuries are suffered as misfortunes, they are not' (Green, 2001). The authors of the ban disagreed: 'Safety experts see injuries waiting to happen as soon as they enter unsafe environments. The challenge is to extend that same sensitivity to all those who control the safety of homes, vehicles, schools, worksites, medical facilities, and other venues where injuries often occur.' This spat goes to the heart of some of the problems facing those wanting to tackle accidental injury. Too much sensitivity to unsafe environments and children are prevented from going on school outings, or even cycling or walking to school alone. Too little and those who are reckless can continue to be so.

Who is most at risk?

- The social, geographical and gender patterning of accidents demonstrate that accidents, and more particularly the distribution of accidents, are not matters of chance; some areas of the country, largely those with significant areas of deprivation, have high accidental injury rates.
- Children in poor housing are at greater risk.
- Boys are at greater risk of accidents than girls.

- Children from large families, or families where there is only one parent to supervise, are more likely to be involved in an accident.
- Child pedestrians are more at risk than children transported in cars. Car transport for some children increases the risk to others.

What doesn't work?

Although this book is about what works, just as important, particularly in the light of spending cuts, is what doesn't work and how to stop doing it. Accident prevention is an area where there remains considerable attachment to ineffective interventions, and to strategies which, in effect, 'blame' parents (in particular mothers) and children, 'educating' them rather than addressing the source of danger.

A common intervention in child accident prevention has been the use of leaflets, posters and pamphlets. A mother in a community study of child injury in Corkerhill, Scotland, suggested that the best use for road safety fliers, which do little more than warn children, the potential victims, to take more care, might be to make them into papier-mâché road bumps. There is little evidence to support the use of educational materials, and some to suggest that it may be hazardous, increasing anxiety among mothers without reducing risks to children (Roberts et al., 1993). A Cochrane review on safety education concludes:

> Pedestrian safety education can result in improvement in children's knowledge and can change observed road crossing behaviour, but whether this reduces the risk of pedestrian motor vehicle collision and injury occurrence is unknown. There is evidence that changes in safety knowledge and observed behaviour decline with time, suggesting that safety education must be repeated at regular intervals. (Duperrex et al., 2002a)

The costs of this kind of intervention are not high, so it might be argued that stopping the provision of printed materials is hardly worth it. A New Zealand study casts a different light on resource allocation (see next box).

The limitations of teaching children to keep themselves safe from traffic

The traditional approach to the prevention of child pedestrian injuries in New Zealand is pedestrian education. However, none of the programmes have been shown to reduce injury rates. The allocation of scarce resources to pedestrian education must therefore be questioned.

A study estimated the number of serious child pedestrian injuries which might be prevented if the resources allocated to pedestrian education were reallocated to approaches such as traffic calming. It was estimated that approximately 18 hospitalisations of child pedestrians could be prevented each year by using this alternative 'treatment', disregarding any other benefits of traffic calming. The results emphasise the need to consider the potential sacrifices involved in the allocation of scarce resources to child pedestrian education rather than to other means of reducing the dangers to children (Roberts et al., 1994).

A good deal of evaluation of strategies and policies in the child safety arena has concentrated on whether or not the message has been received and remembered rather than whether the behaviour of transport planners, motorists or children has changed, let alone whether the child accident rate is affected. The emphasis of road safety work has traditionally focused narrowly on the child's behaviour. Ampofo–Boateng and Thomson's (1989) review of approaches to child pedestrian accidents in the UK suggests that verbal instructions to children can be hazardous when used in isolation. Even when evidence is produced which suggests that health education messages *are* translated into behaviours, the net result does not seem to be a reduction in risk (Roberts and Coggan, 1994). Two before and after studies evaluating the 'Play it Safe' campaign on television aimed at a wide range of possible accidents found no evidence of reduced hospital admissions or reduced use of accident and emergency departments (Williams and Sibert, 1983; Naidoo, 1984).

Even when policies which focus on the potential victims of accidents can be shown to have some impact on children's behaviour, that impact can be short-lived. A Cochrane review (Kendrick et al., 2007) found that home safety education, provided most commonly as a one-to-one, face-to-face intervention in a clinical setting or at home, with the provision of safety equipment, is effective in increasing a range of safety practices. There was no consistent evidence that home safety education, with or without the provision of safety equipment, was less effective in those at greater risk of injury, but the effect of home safety education appeared to diminish with time. Crucially, there was a lack of evidence regarding the impact of these improved safety practices on child injury rates.

What works in making a difference?

Acting on the determinants

The main place of injury for the under-fives is in the home; for the over-fives it is on the road. It has long been established that the determinants of injuries and accidental deaths are multi-factorial (Haddon et al.,1964), though by the time any single death is investigated, there will often be a single explanation – 'speeding', 'drunken driver', 'crossing the road without care'. These explanations, focusing as they do on only one element of the causal pathway, can point in the direction of inadequate solutions (Duperrex et al., 2002a, 2002b), including educational interventions that may attempt to train the public in general, and children in particular, to use the road in the 'right' kind of way. As Walter Morrison, a participant from a low-income community in a high-income country put it in a study of safety as a social value: 'It's like teaching your child to swim in a pool full of alligators' (Rice et al., 1994). Yet children, the most vulnerable members of our society, are frequently allocated the greatest responsibility for dealing with the dangers which may confront them.

In a review of community-based interventions to reduce burns and scalds in children (Turner et al., 2004), only one study showed a significant decrease in paediatric burn and scald injury in the intervention community compared with the controls. The authors suggest that an evidence-based suite of interventions be combined to create programme guidelines suitable for implementation in communities throughout the world. They point out that there remains a gap between 'what we know works' and 'how to make it work' in a real-world setting.

A review of modifications to the home environment (Lyons et al., 2006) was similarly cautious, finding insufficient evidence to determine the effects of interventions to modify home hazards.

Preventing household fires

A review of interventions to promote functioning smoke alarms to reduce injury (DiGiuseppi and Higgins, 2001) describes how many children aged 0–16 are killed or injured by house fires each year, with a steep social class gradient. Fires detected with smoke alarms are associated with lower death rates. The review found that interventions to promote smoke alarms have at most only modest beneficial effects on smoke alarm ownership and function, fires and fire-related injuries.

Carolyn DiGiuseppi went on to lead trials in this area (e.g. DiGuiseppi et al., 2002) which illustrate the dangers of simply deciding 'smoke alarms are good, let's have some'. If money is to be spent effectively, we need to know which smoke alarms will work for whom, and whether at the end of the day, they have the expected effect on the reduction of injuries and deaths from smoke inhalation or burns. Many smoke alarms delivered to households do not get fitted, and many of those that are fitted are disabled because of nuisance alarms or other calls on the battery. How do we make sure they are installed properly, and how do we make sure they are not disabled for causing a nuisance every time the toast is burned? Are some kinds of smoke alarm more likely to be functioning after the passage of time than others? Does it make a difference if the battery has a long life? A Medical Research Council (MRC) funded study explored the effectiveness of different kinds of smoke alarm, combining a randomised controlled trial (RCT) with a qualitative element exploring what the users, installers, recruiters and children of the households in the study area say about their experiences of different kinds of alarm. The MRC's request for a qualitative element to the study was indicative of a growing climate in which the need for different kinds of research to answer different questions is acknowledged. The trial (Rowland et al., 2002) was designed to measure the extent of working smoke alarms in local authority housing in inner London. Nearly half of the alarms installed were not working when tested 15 months later. An editorial at the time of the study publication pointed out that this should lead us to consider the difference between an efficacy trial (what works in perfect conditions) and an effectiveness trial (what works in the real world) (Pless, 2002). Not everyone finds studies of this kind worthwhile. Following publication of the trial results, one reader asked: 'What is … one to make of six pages devoted to the hardly surprising fact that feckless families do not bother to use smoke alarms … The journal is not what it used to be' (Hill, 2002). The feisty response from the editor stressed the importance of context, science and implementation:

> The *New England Journal of Medicine*, published a study showing that the installation of smoke alarms in one area at high risk reduced admissions to hospital and deaths by 80%. This thus seemed to be a highly effective intervention. Authorities around the world might have started offering free smoke alarms to people in deprived areas. But this would not have been sensible after the results of just one study, particularly as the study was not a randomised trial and was undertaken in one particular set of circumstances. The authors of the studies that Dr Hill dismisses thus conducted a rigorous evaluation of whether the intervention would work. It didn't. So now new questions arise. Dr Hill rather gives away his view of the world with the use of the word 'feckless.' I suggest that he tries living for a few months on a very low income in one unheated room with several children in a rough and dangerous area of London. He might discover that 'feckless' is a highly loaded word. (Smith, 2002)

The adults and children in the trial area certainly had reasons other than fecklessness for disabling alarms (Roberts et al., 2004a). The main barrier to smoke alarm use was reported as being the distress caused to neighbours and to children by false alarms. Although trial participants considered themselves to be at high risk from fires, understood the importance of smoke alarm use, and would recommend them to others, their reports suggest that tenants may be balancing fire against other risks to their health and well-being, such as neighbour disputes, when they disable alarms.

Accounts of adverse effects of smoke alarms included:

> '[W]hen that came on I was just like "Oh!" It's such a pitch you just really want to stop it, and in your own home. It's a really calm safe environment and suddenly you've got this, you know, it's screaming at you … you feel completely powerless and that's a horrible feeling in your home, it's something you can't control.' (Adult respondent)

> 'It only went off once, when I burnt something in the kitchen. By that time it had been up for about 8 months. I have a very high ceiling in

the hallway and I'd forgotten how to turn it off. I have a three-year-old daughter, it frightened her so much ... And I didn't know how to turn this thing off.' (Adult respondent)

'I worried about my neighbours. Opposite to me there's an old lady and she can't sleep much and sometimes she sleeps during the day and [the alarm] will bother her.' (Adult respondent)

'Sometimes it's a bit annoying, cos last time I was asleep and my mum was cooking something and then it went on and it was so loud I had to wake up.' (Child aged 10–11 years)

Getting results in the real world, can be complex and difficult. It has to include, as crucial evidence of what to do and how to do it, the contribution of those most directly affected on the receiving end of interventions.

Preventing road traffic accidents and improving the transport environment

- Child pedestrian injury arising from road accidents is a leading cause of accidental death.
- Children in poor neighbourhoods are five times more likely to be injured by a car than those in affluent areas.
- Area-wide traffic calming is designed to control traffic in urban residential areas and has been shown to be effective in reducing child accidents.
- Introducing an area-wide traffic-calming scheme is likely to be an effective measure in reducing inequalities in child health.

Child pedestrian injury arising from road accidents is a leading cause of child accidental death in the UK. However, the number of children injured and killed as pedestrians has fallen over the last 20 years, largely since fewer children walk, as they are taken to school and elsewhere by car. Increased car use is detrimental to children's physical development, increases pollution and also increases the risk to children who do walk or cycle. The poorest children are five times more likely to be killed in a road traffic accident than the best off. Families with fewer resources tend to live in more dangerous housing and road environments, have fewer safe places to play, and go out on foot more often than children from wealthier homes (Hillman et al., 1990; Roberts and Power, 1996).

Use of the car for journeys that would previously have been made on foot has provoked concerns about declining levels of physical activity in childhood and the effect this might have on health in later life. Walking and cycling to and from school, which provided earlier generations of children with regular physical exercise, have correspondingly declined (as indeed have the bicycle parks which used to take up a substantial part of school playgrounds).

It is evident from the reports of interventions which concentrate on addressing individual behaviours that these are likely to have only limited effectiveness, in part because of competing priorities and the law of unintended consequences. Parents driving their child to school may keep their own child safer, but children on foot or on bikes will be put at greater risk as cars zip up to the school gate. The example in the next box shows one of the ways in which risk management replaces one set of risks (cycling to school and having one's parents reported to children's services) with another (lack of exercise).

The dangers of getting safely to school

In 2010, a London couple was reported in the press as having been asked to meet their children's head teacher to be told that unless they supervised their children's bicycle journey to school, they would be referred to Children's Services. There is indeed a risk. There has been a huge decline in children getting to school under their own steam (Hillman et al., 1990) and many are taken to school by car, increasing the injury risk to children on foot and on bikes. Tellingly, a city-wide speed management programme in Gloucester, which included traffic calming, found that at the end of the five-year intervention, the number of parents who said that they let their children go to school on their own had risen from 32% in 1996 to 49% in 2000 (Department for Transport, 2000a).

Two systematic reviews have found that urban traffic-calming schemes can significantly reduce traffic injuries (Elvik, 2001; Bunn et al., 2003). An area-wide scheme implements several changes to traffic across a neighbourhood. It can involve improving main road capacity to carry additional traffic, restricting or removing traffic from residential streets by closing roads, putting in speed humps, roundabouts and chicanes, or introducing one-way systems. Some schemes go one step further by changing the function of the street, prioritising the needs of pedestrians and cyclists over motor vehicles. An initiative of this kind may include the introduction of seating, play areas and increased vegetation, as well as traffic calming, to slow down traffic and make a more social space (Department for Transport, 2000b).

Children themselves identify outdoor safety as important (CYPU, 2002). A report by the Children's Play Council found that 'general fears for personal safety' and 'traffic' were some of the things that stop children from playing outdoors. 'No cars in my street so that I can play outside' (child) (Cole-Hamilton, 2002).

By slowing down traffic, traffic-calming schemes can reduce child injuries from road accidents. The schemes reduce the severity of injury and make it easier for drivers to avoid accidents. Since poorer children are more likely to be injured in a road traffic accident, this is an intervention with the potential to reduce inequalities in child health. Figure 5.1 shows a different kind of traffic calming at a time when there was rather less traffic.

Figure 5.1: Safety device for children crossing the road, Newtown Public School, 5 August 1938

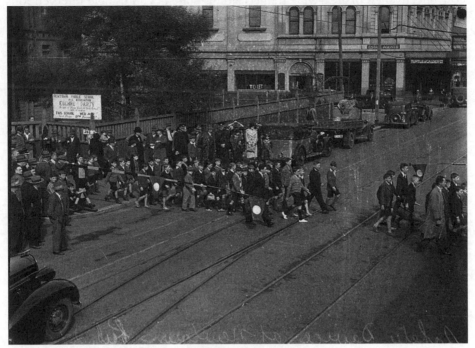

Source: Sam Hood, State Library of New South Wales Collection

The faster the traffic, the greater the risk of death and serious injury. When hit by a car travelling at 40 miles per hour (mph), only one child in 20 will survive. When the car is travelling at 20 mph, 19 children out of 20 will survive. Each one mph reduction in average speed will cut accident rates by 3 to 6% on urban roads, depending on the existing speed and type of road. In 2011, members of the European Parliament called for a 30 km/h speed limit in all residential roads and on single-lane roads without cycle tracks, to help cut the number of children under 14 years old killed by 60% and those seriously injured by 40%. Findings from 200 20 mph zones in the UK indicate that traffic-calming schemes have the potential to be even more effective than they have so far been. When comparing data before and after implementation, child pedestrian accidents fell by as much as 70% and child cyclist accidents by 48% (Webster and Mackie, 1996).

Road accidents have been estimated to cost Britain over £16,000 million a year (Roberts et al., 1994). Traffic-calming measures are likely to have economic benefits in the longer term, both in relation to health and to the environment. A review of speed-limit interventions has reported that stricter enforcement, paired with conversion of junctions into roundabouts, reduces accidents and saves time for drivers, pedestrians and cyclists (Plowden and Hillman, 1996). An economic evaluation of area-wide traffic-calming schemes in England and Wales found that the schemes had the potential to reduce the overall number of accidents by 17,734 accidents a year – a gross annual saving of £357,279,509 (Viudes, 2002). The cost-effectiveness of area-wide traffic-calming schemes and single interventions (for example, speed bumps) depends on the speed limit, the amount of traffic in the area, the inclusion of other speed-reducing initiatives and the relationship between accident-related costs and the costs of setting up a scheme.

Traffic calming has been compared with another popular intervention – road safety education. While the effectiveness of reducing pedestrian injuries from traffic calming has been shown, the beneficial effects on injury reduction from education programmes are less clear (NHS CRD, 1996; Towner et al., 2001; Duperrex et al., 2002a, 2002b). Traffic calming is controversial – and disliked by many motorists. It can have untoward effects, with traffic bumps in some areas being particularly attractive to young motorcyclists and drivers using vehicles which may not be their own. An alternative, also unpopular with many motorists, is the '20 is Plenty' campaign,[1] which, rather than refashioning the street, takes the much simpler approach of encouraging slower traffic. As with many measures for improving the life chances of children, evidence does not translate automatically or without controversy into policy, let alone into the implementation. The disgruntled correspondent below is not atypical of those who resent inconvenience to motorists.

> Website correspondent following the article 'Blackburn and Darwen Health Chief calls for 20mph zones' in *Lancashire Telegraph*, 9 April 2010:
>
> 'It always comes down to the driver doesn't it? Whatever happened to the Green Cross Code? Why have we given up educating children about road safety? Because its easier to target/fine drivers than to blame children in our "think of the cheeeldren" society.'

Drawing on children and parents' safe-keeping strategies – or what are people doing *right*?

We have relatively poor data on how parents manage to keep their children safe most of the time, and why these strategies sometimes fail. But even in high-risk areas, safety is a dominant social value in families, and good practice will draw on this. Towner et al. (1993) reviewed health promotion approaches to child accidents, and their work provides solid evidence that important data on keeping children safe in very localised environments, and strategies for improving the safety of an area, form part of a largely untapped reservoir of knowledge held by ordinary parents and children.

Three observations (Roberts et al., 1995) underlie the contribution which families make to their own safety, and their importance as a source of evidence and experience about what works in reducing accidents to children in unsafe environments:

---

[1] www.20splentyforus.org.uk

—

- **Parents and children living in particular environments are experts in identifying local risks.** Much of the data used by those trying to prevent child accidents are insufficiently localised. Moreover, there are no really robust records of child accidents, only of child injuries. These data tend to describe the consequences of an accident rather than the accident itself and its antecedents. Although people living with local risks may become used to them, and even find ways of avoiding them most of the time, on the whole, they do know what these risks are: the broken fence beside the railway line; the cars that don't stop at the lights even when the green man is showing. Children as young as seven who took part in a Safe School project (CAPT and Roberts, 1993) were able to identify risks and dangers, and suggest practical measures to alleviate them. Effective accident prevention draws on the specialist local knowledge of children and parents.

- **Strategies among parents for keeping their children safe are more apparent than irresponsible risk taking.** Just as local people are well placed to recognise local risks, they are also likely to have strategies for avoiding them, most of which will work most of the time. Prevention policies need to explore the ways in which safety behaviours are integrated into everyday life, and played off against other household routines. (Do I leave my children alone while I go down two floors to hang out my washing, or take them with me down the stone steps?) Effective prevention policies recognise that people living in risky communities are knowledgeable, imaginative and cost conscious and use this expertise.

- **Most accidents occur in hazardous environments.** Spatial and socioeconomic disparities in accident rates are a reflection of differences in the incidence of risky environments. Effective accident prevention is concerned as much with environmental change as with behaviour modification. Road traffic accidents can be 'planned out' of particular urban areas through the use of road layout, chicanes and off-street parking. Other accidents can be reduced by attention to housing design and the provision of safe places for children to play. In practice, between a third and a half of all accidents may be preventable through specific engineering, environmental or legislative measures (Stone, 1993).

Drawing on evidence from the Nordic countries, where the child injury rate is much lower than in the UK, the most promising approaches appear to be those based on the separation of children from traffic and passive measures such as thermostats on water systems preventing scalding.

Child safety and local authorities which consult parents and children

At least one local authority, Rochdale, built the prevention of accidents solidly into their Children's Plan. In order to understand 'what works', the approach they took was to commission research in a part of the town with a high child accident rate. Drawing on the work of Roberts et al. (1995) in Corkerhill, Glasgow, and the expertise of lay people from that community who travelled down to Lancashire to share their expertise, this turned the normal question of what prevents child accidents on its head. Instead of asking why that accident happened, it looked at why there are so relatively few child accidents in areas where there are so many risks. What are parents and children doing right, and how can we learn from it? The next box gives an example of children being involved as active participants in a venture to improve community safety.

Children as experts

In carrying out research into child accidents in Rochdale, Barnardo's was keen to involve children as experts as well as witnesses. In addition to being consulted through group discussions in school, during Child Safety Week a group of schoolchildren conducted their own traffic survey on a main road near the school. They monitored the traffic lights at the school crossing for one hour and found that 31 drivers went through when the lights were red, 73 on amber. The school crossing attendant reported: 'This isn't unusual. I regularly nearly get run over.' One child described an experience which others confirmed: 'the green man was on, and a car just came zooming past and I stopped, and after the car went past, I crossed the road'. In the light of this, their suggestions for improvement were directed towards road planners and drivers, rather than their own behaviour:

'Drivers in Wardleworth have to make their cars slower'
'It would be safer for children by keeping traffic low and police men and ladies walking around'
'You can make a bridge going over the road'

McNeish et al. (1995)

Child protection (non-accidental injury)

An issue as complex as safeguarding and child protection is covered only briefly here. Gilbert et al. (2009a) report that every year, about 4–16% of children are physically abused and 1 in 10 is psychologically abused. During childhood, 5–10% of girls and up to 5% of boys experience penetrative sexual abuse and up to three times this number experience some kind of sexual abuse. A recent *Lancet* series (Gilbert et al., 2009a, 2009b; MacMillan et al., 2009; Reading et al., 2009), National Institute for Health and Clinical Excellence (NICE) guidelines (NICE, 2009) and extensive advice on the Social Care Institute for Excellence (SCIE) and The Centre for Excellence and Outcomes in Children and Young People's Services (C4EO) websites referred to in the Appendix provide some remedy for this deficit. Davies and Ward (2011) and Macdonald (2001a, 2001b) are among high-quality sources of evidence. Below, the discussion is restricted firstly to comparing the response to intentional and unintentional injury, referring back to the discussion in Chapter One of universal and targeted interventions and relating this to smacking, and secondly, to a *Lancet* study with unpromising findings on prevention.

Despite moral panics relating to paedophiles, the danger to life which children face from strangers (other than strangers driving the cars which may run them down) is small. The evidence that could better protect children from this kind of danger is also rather poor. Treatment regimes for adult paedophiles do not have a good record of robust evaluation, and programmes to 'protect' children from predatory and dangerous paedophiles themselves have risky side effects, including a restriction of children's freedom by raising parental levels of anxiety and by providing children with a view that both known and unknown people are unsafe.

Child abuse is not the preserve of any one public or voluntary service, and child protection practices are no longer based on ideas that children suffer abuse predominantly because of the unpredictable action of a few disturbed individuals. Professionals from health, social work, education, police and the law are among those with responsibilities in this area. The differing requirements and knowledge bases of their organisations mean that well co-ordinated action, which benefits individual children at risk of or suffering abuse, and protecting the wider community of children, is fraught with difficulty. This is particularly so given evidence of the sometimes harmful consequences for children and families caught up in child abuse investigations (Cleaver and Freeman, 1995; Farmer and Owen, 1995). Assessing the extent to which there is a social class gradient in child abuse is difficult because of the relatively poor quality of data in this area. There is no one factor associated with abuse that is not also prevalent among families who do not abuse their children (Department of Health, 1995).

Effective interventions in child protection: protecting children from violence

The relative benefits of targeted and universal interventions are discussed in Chapter One. One area where this is particularly salient is in the reduction of physical harm to children. That children have a right to protection and to develop free from violence has been enshrined in the UN Convention on the Rights of the Child. Children have the right to feel safe in their own homes, in the street and the wider environment, and at school (Leach, 1997; Lloyd et al., 1997). Nevertheless, children are afforded a different level of legal protection within families. The law in the UK still permits the use of physical punishment.

While the brutal treatment of children has a long history (Gordon, 1988), it was not until 1962 that an American paediatrician, Henry Kempe, coined the term 'battered baby syndrome' (Kempe et al., 1962) and influenced the identification of a significant problem. Although an essentially medical definition of a syndrome was important in harnessing energy and resources, an approach based on individual psychopathology is only sometimes helpful in dealing with a wide range of damage done to children by the harm which adults can cause, deliberately or otherwise. Hitting small people, according to the current law, is not completely wrong, although teachers are not permitted to hit children and parents are not permitted to hit children hard enough to leave a mark or bruise. UK law is based on an 1860 judgement, where Chief Justice Cockburn stated: 'By the law of England, a parent … may for the purpose of correcting what is evil in the child, inflict moderate and reasonable corporal punishment'.

In 2000, the Department of Health issued a consultation which set out the issue of physical punishment in the context of the government's policy aims and summarised prevailing attitudes. One of the questions asked in relation to the 'reasonable chastisement' defence was:

> Are there any forms of physical punishment which should never be capable of being defended as 'reasonable'? Specifically, should the law state that any of the following can never be defended as reasonable:
>
> • physical punishment which causes, or is likely to cause, injury to the head (including injuries to the brain, eyes and ears)?
> • physical punishment using implements (e.g. canes, slippers, belts)? (Department of Health, 2000, Para 5.7)

In excess of 900 responses were made to this consultation. Unsurprisingly, very few thought the above were reasonable. Some drew attention to the hand or fist also being an implement, and injury to self-esteem and confidence also being significant injuries.

Smacking is first and foremost a human rights issue. But there is no evidence that smacking 'works'. Those countries where smacking is banned in law are not overrun with sociopathic toddlers. There is a strong evidential public health argument, based on Geoffrey Rose's work, which can be mobilised to oppose smacking. Rose and Day (1990) found in samples representing 52 populations in 32 countries that average blood pressure predicted the number of hypertensive people; the average weight the number of obese people; and the average alcohol intake the number of heavy drinkers. Might this also affect other behaviours? Suppose we were to measure how aggressive people are using a rating scale. We might go on to calculate the average level of aggression for the entire population. If we were to plot on a graph people's aggression scores, it would probably show a normal distribution – a few very aggressive people and a few exceptionally inoffensive people at the ends of the scale, with most people in the middle of the range. We condemn frank violence, but fail to discourage in law some kinds of behaviour towards children which falls short of injury. If Rose and Day are right, dealing only with the extremes of aggressive behaviour while ignoring factors which influence aggression in society as a whole is doomed to failure. In the case of violence, it may be more appropriate to focus some of our remedial efforts on 'normal' violence, as well as the extreme, despite the latter being more newsworthy (see Figures 1.2 and 1.3).

We may find, if the Rose hypothesis is correct, that the extent to which we smack our children may be directly related to the prevalence of child abuse. Henry Kempe, who first used the term 'battered baby syndrome' may have been wrong when he suggested that child abuse is the difference between a smack on the bottom and a fist in the face. They may simply be different parts of the same distribution. And if we start to say that a smack is unacceptable, might that change views of slightly more severe smacking, and the smacking that goes a little bit beyond what was intended, and the really nasty thrashing? In other words, the entire distribution of violence towards children could be shifted, and the violent extremes we read of too often in the papers reduced.

Unfortunately, despite the large investment of professional time and resources devoted to the problems presented by parents who provide less-than-adequate care for their children or who abuse them physically or sexually, there are relatively few studies which robustly assess the effectiveness of interventions in this area (Macdonald with Winkley, 2000; Macdonald, 2001a, 2001b; Davies and Ward, 2011). In reviewing the effectiveness literature, where there is a tendency to concentrate on social and psychological variables (social isolation, personal skill deficits), it is important that we do not lose sight of the influence of macro-social variables, including overcrowding, poverty and inadequate resources.

Finally, in relation to prevention, a *Lancet* study looked at the question of whether, once child abuse had been predicted, effective prevention was possible (Lealman et al., 1983). The study ambitiously explored the use of data available at birth to predict abuse, and the effectiveness of supportive measures. In Bradford in 1979, 18% of 2,802 non-Asian infants delivered under consultant care were predicted on the basis of characteristics derived from published studies and from a local retrospective survey, to be 'at risk'. Over the period of follow-up, two thirds of all the recognised abuse in the relevant population occurred in that 18%. Those at risk were allocated to social work/health visiting support. The authors report that those who received greatest attention from social workers and health visitors fared worst. While this study raises more questions and methodological problems than it answers, it is difficult to resist the authors' conclusion that while prediction may be possible, any suggestion that prevention is then straightforward underestimates the complexity of child abuse.

However, we need to remember that the vast majority of children brought up in poverty are cared for by loving families who work hard to protect their children's health and well-being under difficult circumstances and in the face of poor housing, insufficient income and social exclusion (Roberts et al., 1995).

Children are more frequently the victims than the perpetrators of violence (Calouste Gulbenkian Foundation, 1995). Hurting those who are smaller and weaker than oneself is safer than hurting those who are larger or more powerful. The phrase 'What the child needs is ...', is frequently completed, even now, with the phrase 'a good talking to/short sharp shock'. A powerful Children's Society poster suggests: 'What that child needs is a good listening to.'

Key messages

- If we listen to children's views, we often find that 'the environment', 'play' and 'being safe from traffic' are close to the top of their agendas.
- Injury causes a significant number of child deaths in the UK and is an important source of ill health and restriction of freedom for children, and anxiety for parents.
- Pamphlets and safety education have not been shown to be effective in reducing child accidents, and may increase parental anxiety, without addressing the core issues.
- Core issues can be worked on through partnerships with housing and town planners, and transport experts.
- We can learn from children on how they keep themselves safe, and from parents on how they keep their children safe. Treating children and parents as defective in child safety matters is as ineffective as treating airline passengers as defective in air safety matters.
- Smoke alarms are likely to be effective in the reduction of injury through house fires, but only if they are installed and working well.

SIX

What works for vulnerable groups?

Looked-after children and care leavers who are already disadvantaged by the experiences which have brought them into the care system, are further disadvantaged by inadequate evidence of effective interventions, and inadequate use of such evidence as there is.

On the more positive side, in the last few years, a good deal of effort has gone into strengthening the evidence to improve their lives in the here and now, and as the adults they will become. The work of the Social Care Institute for Excellence (SCIE) the National Institute for Health and Clinical Excellence (NICE) the Department for Education (DfE) and The Centre for Excellence and Outcomes in Children and Young People's Services (C4EO) are among those creating, synthesising and using research and other important evidence to underpin effective services.

Despite many poor outcomes for looked-after children, as a Scottish report points out (SWIA, 2006) there is nothing inevitable about their doing less well in education, having poor health or being involved in crime. Looked-after children can overcome adversity in childhood and lead successful adult lives. Relationships with skilled adults and sound support can help looked-after children and young people develop successfully and enjoy stability and the chance to put down roots. There is research-informed evidence for bringing about some of the outcomes which will help looked-after children and care leavers to flourish, but it needs to be understood and used.

This chapter focuses on looked-after children and care leavers – a diverse group at risk of poor health outcomes for whom narrowing inequalities could make a real difference. These children and young people do not constitute a single group. They come into the system with differing backgrounds and differing needs. Some move in and out of the care system; some are in trouble with the law; some are disabled or have long-term medical conditions, some are unaccompanied asylum seekers. Some are parents sooner than they intend to be, or sooner than they can cope with. A high proportion have been maltreated, so successful interventions for any of the difficulties they may face will also need to address the consequences of abuse and neglect (Davies and Ward, 2011).

Using the 1970 birth cohort to look at the outcomes for children who had been in the care system, Viner and Taylor (2005) show that public care in childhood is associated with adverse adult socioeconomic, educational, legal and health outcomes greater than would have been expected simply from childhood or adult disadvantage. Men with a history of public care were more likely to have been homeless, have a conviction, have psychological ill health and be in poor general health. Men but not women were more likely to be unemployed, and non–White ethnicity was associated with even poorer adult outcomes.

Chapter Two describes the need to synthesise data from different sources to look at different questions, or different parts of the same question; demonstrating this, Barn et al. (2005), a study published in the same year as the Viner and Taylor study, used different methods (a survey of 261 young people and 36 interviews) to provide perspectives on the post-care experiences of young people from a range of minority ethnic groups. Their main finding was that the needs of different ethnic groups were very similar. Overall, the experiences of Asian and African young people were generally positive; White, mixed parentage and Caribbean young people faced greater disadvantage. Interestingly, in their study, White young people did worst in terms of placement instability, early departure from care, poor educational outcomes and risk-taking behaviour, including criminal activities. Asian and African young people coming into care in adolescence experienced the least instability in placement and education, and Asian young people reported high levels of satisfaction with their social worker. Asylum-seeking young people were reported to be doing particularly well in their education. Barn et al. were talking to young people aged 16–21; the Viner and Taylor analysis was of cohort study adults. The composition and needs of the population in care have changed over the years, but it is difficult not to draw the conclusion from any of the studies that the individual and social costs of a poor start are high, and that parenting of the state, despite some excellent individual experiences, could be much better.

It is important, however, to avoid any suggestion of determinism which can bring with it low expectations. Happer and her colleagues' (2006) report for the Scottish government takes a refreshing approach in asking young people who had been looked after what helped them to succeed. However poor the start, the future is not set in stone. Children can overcome early experience of trauma and adversity; their histories do not have to predict their futures. They quote Colin:

> 'I'm glad the way my life's turned out. I couldn't wish for any better. If I'd had the perfect family maybe, but I didn't and I can't change that and you know, I'm very happy – very happy when all's said and done.' (Happer et al., 2006)

Likewise some of the children and young people in contact with ChildLine (2011) talked positively of care. One described living with a foster family for the previous two years and of "getting on really well with them; I am happy"; and an 18 year old: "I live in a semi-independent unit. It's like a care home. I'm in my house. I am safe."

A good deal of political and press interest in different family types focuses on the relationship between family formation and particular outcomes. The health and social outcomes for the children of lone, divorced, or gay and lesbian parents is extensively probed. There is a less substantial research literature on the impact of parenting in a different kind of family type – young people brought up in local authority care. Corporate parenting, as it is called, is founded on the principle that a local authority should provide the same support that any good parents would provide for their own children. While a good deal of effort is put into researching the kinds of help that might be given to non-corporate parents in order to help them parent well, with randomised controlled trials (RCTs) and systematic reviews enabling some confidence in the results, more needs to be done to research and trial the quality, extent and enforcement of parenting advice that might be offered to corporate parents.

Although many decisions made by both the state and the great welfare charities in the past would not be made now, there was often an enlightened approach to education, training and health. The Barnardo's children's village in Barkingside, for instance, included a small hospital, and attention was also paid to the wider determinants of health – a decent education, decent employment and a good diet. A photograph in the annual report for 1950 shows children in their hospital beds. The caption reads: 'the education of children like these is one of the more difficult problems of our education adviser ... Every effort is made, however, to give to each boy or girl as much education and as many interests as his or her mental or physical capacity makes possible' (Gilmore, 1950: 21). There were also touching stories of personalised care, and use of the media. Childhood deaths are rarer now than they were 60 years ago. But then, as now, every death of a child was a tragedy. Barnardo's Chief Medical Officer wrote in 1950:

> [the only child who died in the village hospital that year] was a boy of 17 who had been with us for many years, but had been an invalid and spent many weary months in bed because of very bad heart disease. He was gradually getting weaker, and longed to see his father, whom he had not been in touch with for years. We were not able to trace his father's address, so asked the BBC to broadcast an appeal, and the father heard and came to the bedside of his dying boy. To the great joy of the nurses, who had come to esteem his courage, his last days were thus made doubly happy. (Gilmore, 1950:20)

Even earlier, in 1921, Barnardo's Medical Director Dr Albert Carless could write: 'The preventive side of our medical work is really the more important ... in that it touches every child under our charge'. Good record keeping, and joined-up thinking in terms of education and emotional and physical health in children's lives were clearly well understood. Of the child's record, Carless wrote: 'On it are recorded the weight (quarterly) and height (half-yearly), the school standard, the various illnesses of the child. Thus, when the time comes for the child to be prepared for and sent out to its future life, a complete record ... is forthcoming' (Carless, 1921:23).

General health and immunisation

Moving into the twenty-first century, the health of looked-after children and care leavers is a source of concern. They are more likely to have poor physical and mental health (Polnay and Ward, 2000; Richardson and Joughin, 2000) and poor health prospects than the general population. This is not, of course, a simple cause and effect relationship but is mediated by other factors, including pre-care experiences.

Children looked after away from home have extensive unmet health needs (Skuse and Ward, 1999). Of their sample of 249 children from six local authorities, Skuse and Ward found that 54% had unmet physical health needs. For almost two thirds of the children, there were incomplete records on when they last saw a dentist. As Skuse and Ward point out, many of these children enter the care system with pre-existing risks – factors within their home circumstances may mean that they have missed out on health care in the past. They suggest that children looked after may well need compensatory health care, so that immunisations that had previously been overlooked will be given and dental caries treated. A key reason for children looked after away from home having difficulty with adequate health care is likely to be related to moves in care. In their study, only 44% of the children had stayed in the same placement throughout the first year of their care episode, 28% had three or more moves and 15 children had had five or more placements in this period. Those admitted under the age of one had the second highest number of placements (Skuse and Ward, 1999:9).

In a study carried out in Wales (Payne and Butler, 1998), all 593 children looked after by a single local authority on one day were examined. The authors found that looked-after children received poor health supervision, despite formal requirements. In relation to immunisation, looked-after children were significantly less likely to be protected from infectious diseases than other two- to five-year-olds in the community. It was difficult to tell quite how much less likely they were to be protected because records were incomplete. More recently, a study of nine health districts across England, Scotland and Wales showed that 33% of children in public care did not receive the meningococcal C vaccine compared with 15% of children who were living at home and not known to social work services (Hill et al., 2003).

Mental health and emotional well-being

Looked-after children fare disproportionately badly in terms of mental health and emotional well-being. Meltzer et al. (2003) found that among young people aged between 5 and 17 who were looked after by local authorities in England, 45% were assessed as having a mental health problem. In terms of stability, the general health of children seemed to improve as their placement became more secure. About two thirds of children who had been in their current placement for a year or more (67%) were assessed as having very good health, compared with just over half (55%) of those who had been in their placement for less than a year. Children and young people placed out of the local authority area were less likely to receive services from Child and Adolescent Mental Health Services (CAMHS) in their new location.

Figure 6.1 compares children in the looked-after system with children living in private households.

Figure 6.1: Prevalence of mental disorders among 11- to 15-year-olds: looked-after and private household children

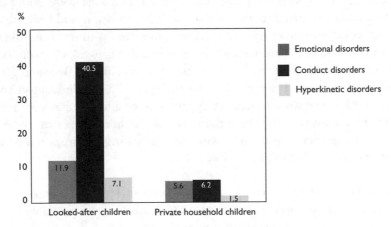

Simkiss, D., reproduced with permission. Based on data in Meltzer et al, (2003). Contains public sector information licensed under the Open Government Licence v1.0.

Data of a different kind were collected from 11- to 17-year-olds who agreed to fill in a self-completion questionnaire reporting on their well-being (Meltzer et al., 2003):

- Children in residential care were more likely than those in foster care to report not spending any time with their friends (13% compared with 3%). Children with any mental disorder were four times more likely than those with no disorder to report not spending any time with their friends.
- Almost a third of the young people were smokers and only 36% had never tried smoking.
- Forty-five per cent of children said they had never had an alcoholic drink. One in twenty children with a mental health problem reported that they drank alcohol almost every day. A quarter of children with an emotional disorder reported drinking at least once or twice a week.

Education

The educational qualifications and subsequent occupations of those who experienced care as children are much poorer than for those brought up in other kinds of household (Cheung and Heath, 1994; Viner and Taylor, 2005). The general research messages about the importance of education for children's and young people's current well-being and later health are set out in Chapter Four. We know that one of the most important things contributing to a good outcome for children after a poor start is education.

In their report on the education of looked-after children, Jackson and Sachdev (2001) examined weaknesses in practice and highlighted promising initiatives. They found that up to 70% of young people in foster care and over 80% in residential care were leaving school with no qualifications; fewer than 20% were going on to further education compared to 68% of the general population, and fewer than 1 in 100 were going to university. Children in care were 10 times more likely to be excluded from school than were their peers and as many as 30% were out of mainstream education because of either truancy or exclusion. Between 50% and 80% were unemployed between the ages of 16 and 25. While Jackson and Sachdev found that social workers frequently failed to see education as a priority, and teachers did not always understand the needs of children in the care system, not every child's experience was poor, with one indicating the importance of having even one stable adult taking an interest:

> 'There was one teacher at my school, he was brilliant. He used to make learning fun and enjoyable. He knew my situation so he probably spoke to me more than anyone in the classroom.'

The problems of moves in care inevitably have an impact on education with children and young people who may be moved to different schools when their placements change, disrupting their education. Children also needed to be in a place where they could learn and do homework in peace.

> 'It's very hard to pass exams if you've got kids running around all night, setting fire alarms off and throwing plates ... The residential care staff let me go up to the office if I needed peace and quiet to study.'

Those in care with babies are likely to need more than the usual chances in life to give their own children better futures, but this does not always happen:

> 'I was only 14 when my baby was born, but no one discussed with me how I could continue my education.'

It is still rare for looked-after young people to take A-levels (or Highers in Scotland) even if their earlier results are good enough. They frequently miss out on careers advice, and some describe how their ambitions are not taken seriously. Figure 6.2 compares the public examination results of those looked after and the general population.

Figure 6.2: Examination results for looked-after children and the general population

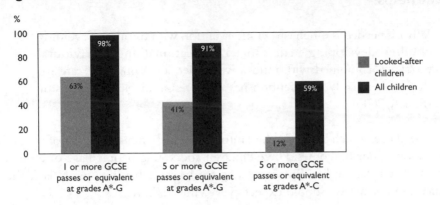

Simkiss, D., reproduced with permission. Based on data in Meltzer et al, (2003). Contains public sector information licensed under the Open Government Licence v1.0.

Settled safe accommodation

Whereas the trend for young people in the general population is for delayed departure from home, or a return to the parental home as young adults, care leavers make an accelerated transition (Biehal et al., 1995; Dixon and Stein, 2002). Having settled accommodation matters to young people leaving care who tend to leave home much sooner than young people in family households.

Jackson and Thomas (1999) point out that when adults or children living in their own family move from one house or community to another, they normally do so in the company of familiar people, and take with them at least some of their furniture and possessions. Even so, there is often a feeling of loss of identity, anxiety and insecurity. Many children who are looked after have an unusually busy life in terms of moves, and do so without the kinds of support the rest of us can normally expect when we move house or job. Some of their difficulties in relation to stability are put into context by looked-after children and young people who telephoned a helpline (ChildLine, 2011):

> 'I feel angry at having to be in care. I feel isolated and sad ... I cannot trust anyone or build relationships as I am moved about so much.' (Sam, age unknown)

> 'I moved into a care home today. I am scared to leave my room. The home is full of other girls who scare me.' (Abigail, aged 16)

> 'I am not feeling good because I am going to get chucked out from my care home. I don't want to move because the care home I am in is nice. I like people in the care home and I like the staff.' (Jacob, aged 15)

What helps?

> What is needed is much earlier intervention with the aim of avoiding children developing major social, educational and behavioural problems, combined with innovative, skilled and consistent care for those where early intervention has not been available or successful. (Polnay, 2000)

The experiences which bring children into the looked-after system are, of course, implicated in poor outcomes. These children and young people have often had a very difficult start in life. But once they are in care, they frequently lack the stability and nurture we should expect every child to have.

What helps in immunisation

Using routine data can work ...

Research can inform development at a local level, and while the 'D' part of R&D may be driven nationally, it is almost always implemented (or not) locally. A well-crafted study of health outcomes for children in care carried out by a consultant in community paediatrics and a social work academic showed lower immunisation rates, more missed medical examinations and poorer general health than for children outside the looked-after system (Payne and Butler, 1998). Their findings were discussed in a peer group comprising both medical and social work staff and young people from the care system, and a number of suggestions made and implemented. These formed the basis for changes in local practice which were then adopted nationally. 'The research resulted in the establishment of the Looked after Children (LAC) nurses here and these are now a standard part of the service UK wide. Our local results showed a major improvement in the immunisation rate and dental care for LAC, to the extent that our local LAC often had a better rate than non LAC children, and also had a far better rate of registration with a dentist, by accessing community dentists, as the availability of NHS dentists is poor.' (personal communication, Heather Payne, 1 August 2011)

But not always ...

While it may often seem worthwhile to intervene on the basis of common sense, the results are not always positive. Ashton-Key and Jorge (2003) performed a simple intervention providing social services with information and advice on immunisation status of looked-after children to see whether it improved uptake. As Figure 6.3 shows, not a single additional child was immunised (signalling, were it further needed, the importance of joint working).

Figure 6.3: Changes in immunisation status of children looked after on 31 March in 1999 and 2000

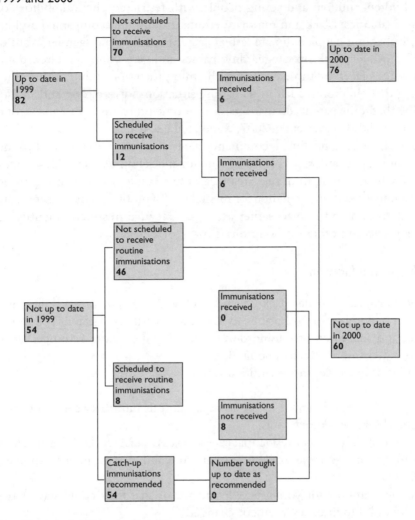

Note: Number of children given in bold.

Reproduced with permission of B M J Publishing Group from Ashton-Key, M. and Jorge, E. 'Does providing social services with information and advice on immunisation status of "looked after children" improve uptake?', *Archives of Disease in Childhood*, 2003, 88, pp 299–301.

What helps in mental and physical health

There are a large number of studies setting out the problems for looked-after children and care leavers and suggesting that something needs to be done; fewer indicate what that might most usefully be. The NICE/SCIE guidance on promoting the quality of life of looked-after young people (2010) found a lack of effectiveness evidence on policies, strategies and interventions that could improve the physical and emotional health and well-being of looked-after children and young people in general and of those who are most vulnerable and disadvantaged in particular. Groups underrepresented in the evidence include babies and very young children, children and young people with restricted physical abilities or learning disabilities, Black and minority ethnic groups, unaccompanied asylum seekers, and young people who are lesbian, gay, bisexual or transgender. Ward et al. (2012), in their book on safeguarding babies and very young children point to the tensions faced by those dealing with child protection, citing both studies indicating that children are left in damaging situations for too long and studies indicating that some parents do manage to overcome problems to provide a good home for a child (Cleaver et al., 2007; Wade et al., 2010).

The NICE/SCIE guidelines recommend that looked-after children and young people should be regarded as a priority group for specialist mental health services, especially when moving from one area to another. While it has been suggested that screening looked-after children for mental health problems could potentially increase detection and lead to earlier access to effective treatment, identifying such treatments and other interventions is more of a challenge.

What helps in education

Better education, better futures (Jackson and Sachdev, 2001) surveyed policy and practice in a number of authorities in England, Northern Ireland, Wales and Scotland, and identified promising developments where extra resources were being allocated and new staff appointed.

Examples of initiatives they identified were:

- structural changes designed to improve communication between education and social services departments;
- training for foster parents, residential care workers, social workers and teachers – aiming to raise awareness of educational issues and increase interdisciplinary working;
- providing transport for young people in care so that they could stay at the same school if their care placement changed;
- developing personal education plans and setting up good educational support for young people in care. Examples of extra help include: revision clubs during the school holidays; extra tuition before exams; paying foster carers to help with reading and homework; and education support projects for unaccompanied asylum seekers in care.

The Department of Education refers to Virtual School Heads appointed to champion the education of looked-after children, and Berridge et al. (2009) evaluated the Virtual School Head pilot schemes in 11 local authorities. These 'heads' do not run schools as such, but have a strategic role raising the profile of the education of looked-after children and working to improve their educational standards as if they were attending a single school. Among the issues they grappled with were deficits in record keeping, and monitoring attendance.

Four of the virtual heads' local authorities piloted private tutoring, about which young people and social workers were generally enthusiastic. Over the period of the pilots, educational statistics on outcomes suggested that they performed well in comparison with other schools, and improvements were at least as good as in the country as a whole, and in some places better. There is currently no statutory requirement for a local authority to have a Virtual School Head for looked-after children. Nonetheless, local authorities have a duty to promote the educational achievement of the children they look after.

A research report for the Scottish government on local authority pilot projects to improve the educational attainment of looked-after children (Connelly et al., 2008) examined pilot projects employing a number of different strategies. The interventions were the provision of direct support (for example, extra tutoring in school or at home); personal education planning; support at transition points in the education system; developing staff and parent capacity to support looked-after children in their education; and using IT and computer-based approaches. Coming to firm conclusions about the effectiveness of these approaches was problematic, since data tracking systems were variable (though the fact that they were being evaluated flagged up what some of the problems were). However:

• attendance at school improved among all the pilot participants;
• exclusion and the number of days excluded fell in the over 15s.

Research into policy and practice in education

In a situation where participation in education and/or training beyond age 16 is increasingly the norm, social background and social support are key influences on who will and who will not take up, and once taken up, make the most of non-statutory opportunities (Dyson et al., 2010; Marmot, 2010).

It is usually a long pathway, both in clinical care and in child public health, from basic R&D to implementation and often the pathway is long for a very good reason – it takes time to do good research (the 'R') and then further time to do the 'D' in terms of sound policy development and implementation. A refreshing example of a speedier process is provided by one piece of research, followed by rapid policy and practice developments (see the next box).

By degrees

In 2004, Buttle UK, a charity which provides financial support through grant-giving programmes to vulnerable children and young people, commissioned an action research project exploring the experiences of the small number of care leavers who go to university. Undertaken at the Thomas Coram Research Unit, 50 care leavers a year entering higher education over three years took part in the research (Jackson et al., 2005). A dissemination programme enabled the trust to ensure that the findings and recommendations had maximum impact.

The project findings influenced government, local authorities, universities and schools to recognise the potential of children in care and provide the support they need to achieve in higher education. Recommendations were included in the Government White Paper *Care matters: Transforming the lives of young people in care* in 2007 and are now incorporated in legislation. Since then, the trust has set up practical support based on the findings, entering into a quality mark arrangement with 88 universities. The quality mark recognises those institutions that go the extra mile both in attracting, recruiting and, crucially, supporting and retaining learners leaving care situations. Since December 2006 the Office for Fair Access has offered specific guidance on support for care leavers including advice on applying for the quality mark. The Frank Buttle Trust and Action on Access have produced a practice guide (Action on Access, 2010) to be used to inform institutions yet to apply for the quality mark, as well as to consolidate the practice of those which already have it.

Building on this, the trust has recently run 18 pilot schemes to extend the quality mark into further education, with a view to informing a trustees' discussion on rolling out this programme. Buttle UK also has a student and trainee grants programme which awards financial support to young people in difficulties to help them attend further education and training. By funding course costs, equipment, field trips or basic day-to-day living costs, the charity relieves the financial pressures and worries that often force vulnerable young people to abandon their studies early. This may be particularly relevant to young people who are vulnerable, since at the end of 2010, 141,800 (7.3%) 16- to 18-year-olds were not in education, employment or training (NEET) (Department for Education, 2011).

What helps in housing

A review carried out for C4EO (Stein, 2010) provides evidence-informed key messages on what works in increasing the number of care leavers in 'settled, safe accommodation'. For young people themselves, being in safe, settled accommodation is a top priority on leaving care and is about where they live, rent that is affordable, and being helped in budgeting and in managing their accommodation. Other key messages include:

- Being in 'settled, safe accommodation' is associated with increased well-being and engagement in education, employment or training.
- Young people are likely to be in such accommodation after leaving care when they (i) have good-quality care which provides them with stability and pays attention to their education and well-being and (ii) are supported to leave care gradually, at an older age.
- It is important to identify groups at particular risk of poor housing outcomes early on, including young people with social, emotional and behavioural problems; young disabled people who do not meet the threshold for adult services; and young asylum seekers.

- Housing and children's services need to identify problems with accommodation early on, have clear contingency arrangements, including sufficient emergency accommodation to prevent homelessness, and have specialist accommodation for young people with higher support needs.

While the adverse effects of early parenthood, and in particular early motherhood, are more frequently reported than positive findings, a small-scale qualitative study of supported housing for young people leaving care in Wales (Hutson, 1997) suggested favourable outcomes in terms of stability and maturity for those who were early mothers. Despite the enormous challenge of having and looking after a baby, the young women she spoke to seemed more closely drawn into mainstream life. One young mother in Hutson's research (1997:49) got up at six o'clock every day, got herself and her two-year-old daughter ready and caught the bus at eight to a college 10 miles away. With her daughter in the crèche, she studied. While parenthood before or shortly after leaving care is unlikely to be the best start to life (as a baby) or adult life (as a mother or father), optimal support in the early years for those who do become parents, and for their children, is likely to be effort well invested.

Housing and health

Barnardo's made the link between care leavers' poor housing and a range of poor health outcomes, and has done something about it. For many years, Barnardo's Marlborough Road project in South Wales has provided a range of services related to health, education and supported housing:

- All young people and children who come into the supported housing projects are either taken to or encouraged to register with a GP and dentist. Ninety per cent are registered.
- Cooking sessions are held at Cardiff Young Families Project. Young people are encouraged to cook healthy food for themselves and others from scratch. Most reported that they enjoyed sitting down at a table together and cooking a healthy meal as a team.
- In the supported housing project for single young people, 95% of young people are on training courses. The remaining 5% are planning with support workers to access training within the next year.
- A support service for young parents offers three groups a week for young women who are either pregnant or have children. The service offers support with parenting, learning opportunities and formal certificated courses.
- Most of the young women have a learning portfolio by the time they finish the support service for young parents.

Barnardo's (2008–09)

Work

Many young people starting out in life can get a chance from friends or family to work shadow, or go to work with their mums or dads. Fewer young people brought up in the care system have these opportunities. But if the state is your mum and dad, you are being parented by a major employer. This means that there are opportunities to be used.

Islington Career Start

Since 2005, Islington Career Start has provided ring-fenced job opportunities and work placements for looked-after young people and care leavers. The scheme provides access to a range of opportunities, including work experience, work shadowing, permanent jobs, temporary jobs and apprenticeships. The scheme also organises information sessions focusing on a range of different careers, employer visits and workshops.

Permanent and temporary jobs identified as suitable for the scheme are advertised to the entire leaving care cohort (16- to 24-year-olds). The scheme has initiated an additional stage to the recruitment process – a one-month unpaid work trial, so that young people who perhaps lack confidence in selling themselves have the opportunity to prove themselves on the job.

The manager cautions:
'Employability skills do not suddenly exist once a young person reaches statutory school leaving age. Councils need to provide young people with opportunities at an early age that will encourage them to develop confidence in their own abilities and will help them identify and develop useful employability skills.'

The scheme is being evaluated by the Centre for Child and Family Research, Loughborough University.

Smith (2010)

Children and young people with complex needs

In England, the Department for Education identifies a group of children in the looked-after category as needing very specialist and expensive services to meet their complex needs. The Department is piloting services which include the following.

The Family Drug and Alcohol Court (FDAC)

There has been a good deal of important work on the impact of drug-using parents on the well-being of their children (Barnard, 2003, 2005a, 2005b; Barnard and McKeganey, 2004) and the kinds of interventions which make a difference to families in trouble (Forrester and Harwin, 2011). Parental substance misuse is a major risk factor for child maltreatment and family separation and for poor educational performance and substance misuse by children and young people. In cases where parental substance misuse is a key element in local authority decisions to bring care proceedings, a new process is being piloted at a London Family Proceedings Court. This is a problem solving court which involves both legal care proceedings and a therapeutic approach. The FDAC specialist team, which includes drug and alcohol treatment specialists, nurses and social workers, provides intensive assessment, support, interventions and co-ordination of care for families affected by parental drug and/or alcohol misuse. A judge works closely on the case, playing a very active motivational role, though one where lapses are openly addressed. Judges are trained in motivational interviewing, with two dedicated district judges on the scheme – giving a greater likelihood of the same judge throughout. This differs from the normal procedure, which may lack continuity, where there is no specialist team attached to the court and where assessments may be ordered from a range of experts and take months to be carried out and reported. As a court officer quoted in Munro (2003) put it, 'If we lose time, for whatever reason ... we are losing part of a child's childhood that we can't get back.' The main aims of the project are:

- to test out whether the FDAC model improves outcomes for children, in terms of either rehabilitation or earlier placement outside the family if parents fail to engage;
- to determine whether more timely decision making for the most vulnerable children takes place;
- to see whether parents are successful in controlling or giving up their substance misuse and whether there is greater engagement and retention with substance misuse services. The aim is to get parents engaged with services and not to go through a range of assessments;
- to increase the court's confidence in making decisions without the need for reports from a wide range of external experts. The aim is for fewer requests for expert reports and fewer repeated assessments.

The evaluation team (Harwin et al., 2011) point out that while a small-scale study can make only tentative suggestions about what lies behind the results, their findings show this to be a promising approach with a higher rate of mothers addressing substance misuse, and speedier family reunification or placement. The Nuffield Foundation has funded further evaluation on a larger sample to establish whether FDAC continues to show better child and parent outcomes at final order than in comparison cases heard in ordinary care proceedings. The researchers will also look at whether children return to or remain with parents and whether the positive outcomes are sustained once FDAC's involvement ends.

Family group conferences and kinship care

Somewhat more problematic in terms of the evidence are family group conferences. A Scottish review (Barnsdale and Walker, 2007), while generally positive about process issues, including the willingness of families to come together and plan, reports that in some studies, children and young people did not feel heard. They point out that there have been more studies on process issues than on plan implementation and outcomes for children. Those that there have been suggest that the process can falter because either the family or social work services fail to meet their commitments. In comparing outcomes from different studies, Marsh and Crow (1998) and Lupton and Nixon (1999) were somewhat more positive, finding only that outcomes for children were no poorer than traditional decision making. In-depth interviews of kinship care in one London borough (Broad et al., 2001) found the young people they interviewed overwhelmingly positive about their experiences, mentioning feeling loved, settled and safe. Negative aspects reported included restrictions to their freedom, and financial difficulties. Kinship carers were also very positive, highlighting their love for the young people, and for the grandparents, a wish to support their children. However, half of them were struggling to cope with the behaviour of the young people, and reported problems in relation to money, loss of freedom, and overcrowding.

Potentially worrying, however, are findings from a Swedish study for which the abstract is reproduced in full below. This work is somewhat similar to the mentoring example in Chapter Four. This is an idea which looks as if it might work and we can all see why it might. It is heart-warming that people want to step in and lend a hand, and it is not too complicated to make sense. However, both positive findings from some studies, and the less positive findings (see box below) throw into sharp relief some of the problems described in Chapter Two on methods of assessing what works. People are often very willing to report in an interview or survey that they are happy with services, particularly if they have been treated decently; by the very nature of this intervention, it is likely that those concerned will report better communication and that children will not need to be accommodated so often. What we are unlikely to find through these methods is what the outcomes in terms of a child's safety and medium- and long-term well-being might be.

A three-year follow-up of family group conferencing in Sweden

Objective: Between 1995 and 1997, the Swedish Association of Local Authorities implemented Family Group Conferences (FGC) in 10 local authorities throughout Sweden. This study reports on client outcomes of this implementation.

Method: Ninety-seven children involved in 66 FGCs between November 1996 and October 1997 were compared with 142 children from a random sample of 104 traditional child protection investigations by the Child Protective Services (CPS). All children were followed for exactly three years for future child maltreatment events reported to CPS. Effects were modelled using multiple regressions, controlling for the child's age, gender, family background, and type and severity of problems.

Results: After controlling for initial differences, FGC-children experienced higher rates of re-referral to CPS compared to the group that had been processed in traditional investigations. They were more often re-referred due to abuse, were more often re-referred by the extended family, were longer in out-of-home placements, but tended over time to get less intrusive support from the CPS. FGCs were not related to re-referrals of neglect, of case-closure after three years or number of days of received services. The results suggest that the impact of the FGC was scant, accounting for 0–7% of the statistical variance of outcome variables.

Conclusions: The findings did not support the alleged effectiveness of the FGC model compared to traditional investigations in preventing future maltreatment cases. If these results are confirmed in future research, they serve as a reminder of the necessity to evaluate models based on untested theories or on extrapolations from other countries/cultures, before these models are widely spread in a national practice context.

Reprinted with permission from Elsevier Science from Sundell, K. and Vinnerljung, B. (2004) 'Outcome of family group conferencing in Sweden: a 3 year follow-up', Child Abuse and Neglect, 28(3), pp. 267–87.

Key messages

General
- While it is never too early to make a difference to the lives of young people, and early life is the best time to intervene effectively, it is never too late.
- The desire to 'do something' can mean that interventions with vulnerable groups are not properly thought out and may be ineffective or worse.
- There are some promising approaches which deserve more serious evaluation.
- Promising interventions and associated evaluations need to be planned and discussed with vulnerable people on the receiving end of services.
- The imperative to be innovative undermines the use of the best available evidence. There is a middle way, building on the best available evidence, and robustly testing the next steps.

Looked-after children and care leavers
- Looked-after children and young people should have clear expectations for their care and well-being (Children's Rights Director for England, 2007) and expect to take part in decisions that affect their lives, be kept healthy and safe, be treated with respect, and be treated equally to other children and young people.
- Despite increased attention to this area, looked-after children and care leavers can still get a poor deal from services, rather than the concentrated effort needed to repair some of the damage which brought them to the looked-after system in the first place.

- Where there are well-validated interventions, they should be used. We need to use the best of what we already know as well as creating new knowledge.
- Where interventions are not well-validated, they are, in effect, experiments and should be robustly tested to make sure they are doing more good than harm.

SEVEN

Tackling the causes of the causes

The difficulty with single behavioural interventions in addressing the effects of poverty and other disadvantages on health, even when they are evidence-informed, is that they are the ambulance at the bottom of the cliff rather than the fence at the top. Even programme interventions, some more evidence-based than others, are no alternative to confronting the reality that inequalities in health can be fundamentally tackled only by policies that tackle broader inequalities. This means a society which is less unequal – something which has a degree of public support in the UK (Park et al., 2011).

In recent years, there have been a number of policy reports on inequalities in health, many of whose recommendations are directed at child health in particular and/or reducing childhood poverty. A formal recognition of the fundamental problem of child poverty and the need to combat it is now enshrined in legislation in the UK. Policies and practices beyond the individual level including in housing, employment and transport, as well as taxation, are more likely to have a positive effect at a population level than any number of interventions directed (for instance) towards individual parents.

Children and young people are both users of health care and providers of care to themselves and others. No policy to address inequality can ignore the children as actors themselves, rather than objects of concern who are simply recipients of care. Unless children are at the heart of policy, their interests are unlikely to be prioritised other than at the level of rhetoric. Children are not small adults. If we are to reduce inequalities in health, we need to provide services which recognise their needs as children.

The road to wisdom

The road to wisdom?
– Well, it's plain
and simple to express:
Err
and err
and err again
but less
and less
and less.

Piet Hein (1905–96)

Inequalities in child health

Piet Hein, the Danish physicist, mathematician and poet starts and finishes this book. The brief poems which he started to write for a newspaper when his country was occupied by Nazis are said to have conveyed hidden messages to the Danes. They provide a serious message without being solemn. Now out of print, there is something hopeful about them.

If there is anything positive and hopeful to be said about inequalities in child health, it is that they show that things do not have to be the way they are, nor need we wait until everything can be done before anything can be done (Mitchell, 1984).

Risks for poor health outcomes are cumulative and the benefits of early intervention cannot be underestimated, but even when individual or community-level interventions to improve health are successful, they cannot entirely override the fundamentally disabling effects of poverty and inequality and overcome socioeconomic disadvantage (Power and Hertzman, 1997). Providing opportunities to disadvantaged children will improve their life chances, but will not put them on an even playing field with their more advantaged peers. Practice interventions rely very largely on behavioural change (of practitioners or service users rather than of politicians, policy makers and planners), and as Davey Smith et al. (1990:376) argue, 'intervention becomes reduced to developing culturally sensitive methods for encouraging changes in lifestyle, and neglects changes in the environment'.

Internationally

This book is directed towards those tackling inequalities in health in wealthier nations. Collison et al. (2007) drawing on data on wealthy nations from the 2003–06 State of the World's Children reports (UNICEF, 2003, 2004, 2005, 2006) demonstrate that strong associations between income inequality and child mortality persist.

Global inequalities in relation to low- and middle-income countries are, of course, even more stark. Worldwide, almost 9 million under-fives die annually (Black et al., 2010), and Viner et al. (2011) show that adolescents and young adults have benefited less than younger children from the epidemiological transition.

According to the WHO (2008) at the launch of *Closing the gap* (CSDH, 2008):

> a girl in Lesotho is likely to live 42 years less than another in Japan. In Sweden, the risk of a woman dying during pregnancy and childbirth is 1 in 17400; in Afghanistan, the odds are 1 in 8.

They point out that biology does not explain any of this. Instead, the differences between – and within – countries result from the social environment where people are born, live, grow, work and age.

Closing the Gap's core recommendations are to:

- improve daily living conditions, including the circumstances in which people are born, grow, live, work and age;
- tackle the inequitable distribution of power, money and resources – the structural drivers of those conditions – globally, nationally and locally;
- measure and understand the problem and assess the impact of action.

In terms of the more effective and equitable use of resources, NICE International is increasingly playing a role at the invitation of other countries. And in terms of crises and disasters, where the desire to 'do something' can be overwhelming, the Cochrane Collaboration Evidence Aid project[1] seeks to highlight which interventions work, which don't and which, no matter how well meaning, might be harmful.

While it is sometimes assumed that health advice to poorer countries, or poorer people in richer countries, is the prerogative of the better off, the wealthier world has a good deal to learn from low-income countries in terms of low-impact low-cost policies and practices. This is the case in relation, for instance,

Figure 7.1: Mean income inequality ratio and under-five mortality rate in wealthier OECD countries

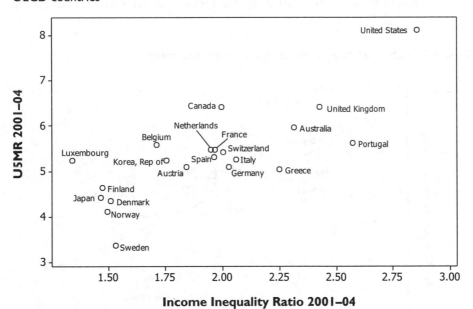

Income Inequality Ratio 2001–04

Note: U5MR = Under-five mortality rate.

Reprinted with permission of Oxford University Press; from Collison, D., Dey, C., Hannah, G. and Stevenson, L. 'Income inequality and child mortality in wealthy nations', *Journal of Public Health*, 2007, doi. 10.1093/PUBMED/FDM009

---

[1] www.cochrane.org/cochrane-reviews/evidence-aid-project

to the approach taken to happiness and well-being in Bhutan and in terms of a technology as easily transportable as happiness, Kangaroo Mother Care (KMC), the major component of which is skin-to-skin contact between mother and baby (Conde-Agudelo, et al., 2011).

Context

Towards the end of the twentieth century, the preferred government term for inequalities in health in the UK was the somewhat loaded 'health variations' (though the weasel words did not prevent an Economic and Social Research Council programme of that name producing important and influential work).

In the UK, there has been an impressive number of government and other enquiries and reports over the last 30 years or so touching on both inequalities and child health. Rather than report their findings here, some are referred to in the Appendix. The approach taken in this chapter is to outline the importance of both 'big' and localised policy in tackling the determinants of inequalities in child health and to provide some examples.

More egalitarian societies tend to have higher, sometimes much higher, standards of health than those that are less equal, as Wilkinson (1994) and Wilkinson and Pickett (2009) have shown. Figure 7.2 demonstrates this, using

Figure 7.2: Child well-being is better in more equal rich countries

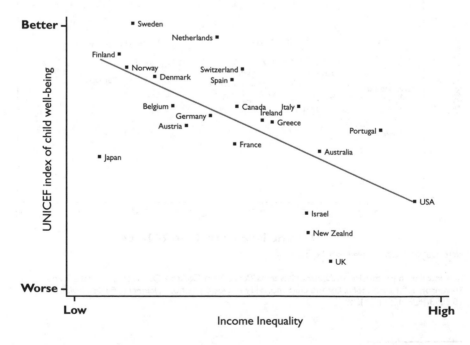

Figure reproduced with permission. *Source:* Wilkinson and Pickett, *The spirit level,* Penguin (2009)

UNICEF's composite measure of child well-being, to show Finland, Norway, Denmark and Sweden all doing well, and the US (from where many of our policy ideas are derived) doing rather badly. The story of Nordic success using the more traditional infant mortality index is much the same as Figure 7.1 shows. Educational achievement shows Finland topping the charts. In terms of bullying, fighting and 'finding peers not kind and helpful', the Nordic countries come out well, and the US, UK and Portugal poorly.

Poverty

The commitment in the UK to take children out of poverty by 2020 is probably the single most important long-term policy in reducing both the gap and the gradient in health. Getting this into legislation in 2010 was a major achievement. It reflects the fact that some things can be done only by governments, but as Sutherland et al. (2008) point out, it will be virtually impossible for the government to end child poverty if payments to families with children rise more slowly than other incomes.

While the growth of inequality has been accompanied by increased research and policy interest in the poor, as Orton (2006) points out, we also need to understand more about the wealthy. Social attitudes towards inequality are ambivalent, with most people recognising and (to an extent) deploring inequality, but with little consensus on what should be done about it. On the whole, people appear to think that those on higher incomes are paid too much rather than that those on lower incomes are paid too little (Orton and Rowlingson, 2007a, 2007b). In the recent British Social Attitudes report (Rowlingson et al., 2010) it was reported that:

- 78% think the gap between those with high incomes and low incomes is too large, up from 73% in 2004. Income inequality is seen as having negative impacts;
- 80% say children from better-off families have many more opportunities than children from less well-off families.

However, in terms of what might be done, people are more ambivalent (Sefton, 2005). When people were asked specifically whether the government should take measures to redistribute income, the largest proportion (38%) thought that the government was doing too little or much too little in terms of redistribution from the best off to the less well off. Thirteen per cent thought that the government was doing too much in that direction, 28% about the right amount, and 20% found it impossible to say. The term 'redistribution' appears to have an effect on the way in which the people view inequality and income, with, as Orton and Rowlingson show, a far higher percentage thinking that the gap is too great than thinking that the government is doing too little about it. Figure 7.3 describes those saying that the inequality gap is too large, too small and about right.

Figure 7.3: The income gap is too large/too small/about right

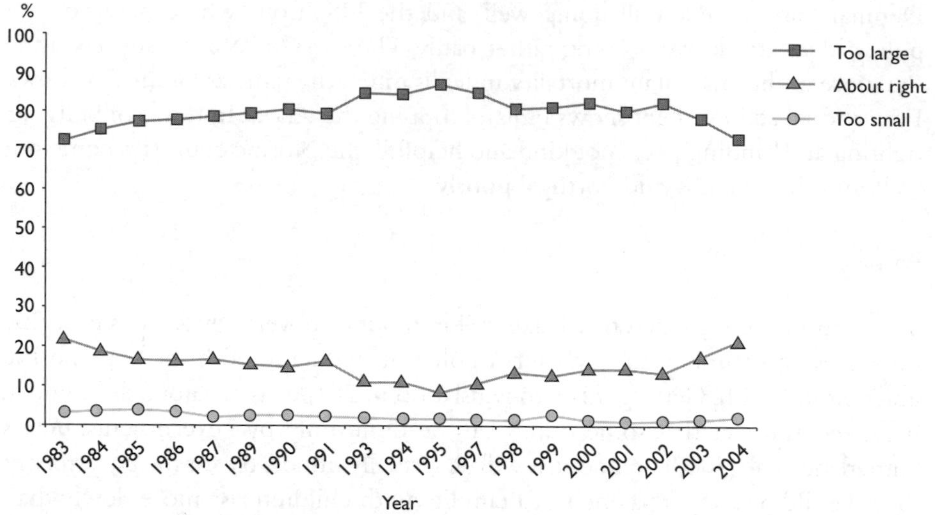

Source: Orton and Rowlingson (2007a, figure 1, p 10)
Reproduced by permission of the Joseph Rowntree Foundation

Policies for directly addressing inequalities in child health

There may be no medical or scientific intervention to cure inequalities in health, but there have been real gains. As with so much else in public, social and fiscal policy, there is no magic bullet, but rather a range of strategies which need to respond to what the evidence suggests about how to bring about beneficial change.

The 20 years within which government ministers originally pledged to take children out of poverty in the UK from 2000 was a short time in policy terms, but a long time in the life of a child. Fundamental problems require long-term solutions. In the meantime there are a range of policies which address inequality in the current health and well-being of children.

One issue frequently raised by those of all political colours is that of universal and targeted services, benefits or interventions. Should child benefit be an entitlement for all, or only for some? Should services be provided for all, or only in areas of deprivation? The problem with a targeted model of intervention is that not all disadvantaged children conveniently live in disadvantaged communities. Most do not. Day care and early years provision need to be addressed through a universal service, just as education and health are, if they are to reach all of those in need. The relative lack of effectiveness of area-based policies has been well documented for over 25 years (Shaw et al., 1999:177). The weight of the evidence is that policies are most effective when applied to the whole society, and that targeting particular groups with training, advice or counselling may do less good than expected.

It is unlikely that any intervention aimed at changing individual behaviour, however well designed and carefully implemented, will significantly reduce inequalities in health at a population level, partly because of the more enthusiastic take-up of opportunities to benefit health and well-being by those who are already better off. This is unlikely to change significantly so long as the policy direction in health remains antipathetic to regulation and legislation, despite the strong track record that such measures have in bringing about cultural change and health benefits. When seat belt legislation was introduced in the UK in the 1980s, it was unpopular; similarly with wearing a motor cycle helmet and breathalysers to detect drink driving. Until the penalties and campaigns against drinking and driving started to have an effect, 'one for the road' had tended to be considered a hospitable rather than a homicidal offer.

Those antipathetic to anything that might be considered 'nanny state' hold that the behaviour for which individuals are themselves directly responsible is the most crucial thing to address. The publication of *Nudge* (Thaler and Sunstein, 2008) has been hailed by some as an example of leading people to do the right thing by guile rather than force. In an article called 'Judging nudging', Marteau et al. (2011:342) write: 'the appeal of nudging is self evident: it proposes a set of seemingly simple, low cost solutions that do not require legislation ... [This] holds particular appeal for governments and others wanting a smaller role for the state in shaping the behaviour of its citizens.' The authors provide examples of the ways in which we can be nudged into health-damaging behaviours by, for instance, neighbourhood design which is friendlier to cars than to pedestrians or cyclists. While by no means hostile to the idea that there may be circumstances where the 'nudge' approach could improve public health at a population level, they warn that without regulation to limit the potent effects of unhealthy nudges in environments shaped largely by industry, nudging towards healthier behaviour may struggle to have an effect. This is reinforced by a series of articles in the *Lancet* which underline the argument that dealing with obesity, for instance, is complex, involving strong vested interests. Swinburn et al. (2011) advocate action on supply-side measures, and an editorial and commentaries in the same issue of the journal appear to concur:

> Governments' reactions so far are wholly inadequate and rely heavily on self-regulation by the food and beverage industry, and the so-called nudge approach ... The UK Government, in particular, has made it clear that only voluntary agreements with food and beverage companies are on the agenda, and many of the public health committees are made up of large numbers of these very industry representatives.

Asking the crucial question, 'do these voluntary agreements work?' they respond 'All indications so far are that they do not' (*Lancet*, 2011). Table 7.1 provides examples of nudging and regulating actions.

Table 7.1: Examples of nudging and regulating actions

	Nudging	Regulating
Smoking	Make non-smoking more visible through mass media campaigns communicating that the majority do not smoke and the majority of smokers want to stop	Ban smoking in public places
	Reduce cues for smoking by keeping cigarettes, lighters, and ashtrays out of sight	Increase price of cigarettes
Alcohol	Serve drinks in smaller glasses	Regulate pricing through duty or minimum pricing per unit
	Make lower alcohol consumption more visible through highlighting in mass media campaigns that the majority do not drink to excess	Raise the minimum age for purchase of alcohol
Diet	Designate sections of supermarket trolleys for fruit and vegetables	Restrict food advertising in media directed at children
	Make salad rather than chips the default side order	Ban industrially produced trans fatty acids
Physical activity	Make stairs, not lifts, more prominent and attractive in public buildings	Increase duty on petrol year on year (fuel price escalator)
	Make cycling more visible as a means of transport, for example, through city bike hire schemes	Enforce car drop-off exclusion zones around schools

Reproduced with permission of BMJ Publishing Group; from Marteau et al. (2011) 'Judging nudging: can nudging improve population health', *British Medical Journal*, 342: doi:10.1136/bmj.d228.

Area-based regeneration

Addressing problems one symptom at a time can lead to surprising contradictions. A review of UK area-based regeneration initiatives for instance, showed some improvements in average employment rates, educational achievements, household income and housing quality, all of which may contribute to a reduction in inequalities in health, but it also noted that these can be accompanied by an increase in housing costs which renders residents poorer, and the original residents may leave the area (Thomson et al., 2006).

This was the case in Corkerhill, the community referred to in Chapter Five, which became a WHO 'Safe Community'. Better housing was the coveted prize for the tenants there, and some time after the completion of the Safety as a Social Value study there in the 1990s, this did indeed occur. The new housing brought benefits for some tenants but many others were decanted out to other places and never returned. In that sense, they did get what they asked for – new housing – but at a price too high for the population in residence at the time. One resident influential in the local research, Betty Campbell, explained:

'The likes of myself, you see it firsthand. The houses aren't built with people in mind – not the people who were living here in the tenements. They got moved out. They're here, there and everywhere now. [The houses] weren't supposed to be buy-to-let ... They were meant to be affordable.'

There is now mixed tenure housing, and although by UK standards, prices of houses with the garden that every parent on the estate had yearned for are well below the national average, they are also well beyond the reach of many. 'Buy to let' ownership has meant less community engagement and solidarity (Roberts et al., 2010).

Housing

Children from low-income families are more likely to live in poor housing and have fewer safe places to play (Roberts et al., 1996; HM Treasury, 2004a, 2004b, 2008). However, injury is not the only negative heath outcome associated with poor housing and overcrowding. Other problems include respiratory difficulties, developmental delay, poor sleep patterns and exposure to other hazards, including crime.

In order to argue for decent housing, it should not be necessary to 'prove' the health effects of poor housing; it is a rights issue. However, good-quality studies indicate the health effects of poor housing. Platt et al. (1989) showed a strong correlation between the degree of dampness, mould and air spores and a wide range of symptoms. Hyndeman (1990), looking at housing in Tower Hamlets found a close correlation between dampness/mould and respiratory symptoms, diarrhoea, vomiting, depression and general ill health. In terms of housing design, it has been estimated that 11% of home accidents to children were associated with unsafe architectural features (DTI, 1995). A survey of houses in multiple occupation in 1985 showed that four out of five required statutory action to deal with inadequate means of escape from fire (Kirby and Sopp, 1986).

New Zealand researchers (Howden-Chapman et al., 2007) found significant improvements in health-related quality of life in a randomised controlled trial (RCT) of home insulation, and concluded that targeting home improvements at low-income households significantly improved social functioning and physical and emotional well-being (including respiratory symptoms). A further study (Howden-Chapman et al., 2008) indicated the role of adequate heating systems in improving asthma symptoms and reducing days off school.

According to Thomas and Dorling (2004), in the previous 10 years, the 'housing wealth' per child in the 10% best-off areas had risen 20 times more than in the worst-off areas. Ten years earlier, an average house price in Kensington would buy two houses in Leven, Fife. In 2004, it could buy 24. The researchers argued that a slowdown in housing wealth would be unlikely to have substantial impact on this inequality. Housing wealth gives families greater security and opportunity, and families who do not have this cannot earn their way out of this early disadvantage.

Roads and the wider environment

There is huge potential for savings in relation to child injury, but further evidence is required on the cost and effectiveness in this area (Holtermann, 1995:129). A particular problem here, as in a number of other areas, is that savings do not necessarily accrue to the government department incurring costs. Across a range of accidents to children, changing the environment is one of the most effective ways of achieving greater safety. Product improvements have also led to accident reductions, and child-resistant packaging of medicine and other hazardous materials have led to a steep reduction in poisonings. A review by Towner et al. (1993) looked at the effectiveness of health promotion in the reduction of accidents, broadly including education, environmental modification and legislation. In the case of traffic accidents and the environment which children have to negotiate outside the home, they found no evaluated studies on the use of the law to make drivers more responsible for their actions.

Reducing the speed limit reduces death on the road, and where injury occurs, it is less serious (Pilkington, 2000). A London study indicates that putting 20 mph zones in more deprived areas has helped mitigate widening inequalities in road injury (Steinbach et al., 2010). In countries where children and traffic are separated, children ride bicycles, walk and play with a lower likelihood of injury. There are few policy areas where a simple decision can have immediate consequences for children's welfare, but reduction of road traffic speed is one such issue. There is also, unfortunately, evidence that the very substantial decline in child accident rates in the last 30 years has been gained primarily at the expense of children's freedom to roam and tendency to lead more sedentary lives. The consequences for children include poorer physical health due to lack of exercise, reduced social networks, less independence and greater demands on parental time to escort children to school.

Natural environment and well-being

Green space, use of the natural environment and having safe places to play all have an impact well beyond reducing injury (Lester and Maudsley, 2006; Bird, 2007). Improved local environments are reported to have a positive impact on social cohesion and interaction, with streets where the traffic is light associated with more social contact and larger geographical areas for which people feel responsible.

In 2008, the National Institute of Health and Clinical Excellence (NICE) produced the first national, evidence-based recommendations on how to improve the physical environment to encourage physical activity to improve health. While not specifically directed at children, the recommendations impact on the environments in which children grow up and their parents live and work. They also chime in well with children's frequently reported view that climate change is the key issue for the future. The NICE recommendations are not only for the National Health Service (NHS) and local authorities, but for all who have a role or responsibility for a built or natural environment, including planners, transport authorities, building managers, designers and architects. The recommendations most applicable to children and young people include:

- ensuring that planning applications for new developments always prioritise the need for people (including those whose mobility is impaired) to be physically active as a routine part of their daily lives;
- ensuring that pedestrians, cyclists and users of other modes of transport that involve physical activity are given the highest priority when developing or maintaining streets (NICE, 2008c).

A further advantage to some of these measures is that they also have the potential to reduce our carbon footprint. Doing something about global warming is a priority for children.

This and other work on interventions to improve health and reduce inequalities suggest that efforts be made to strengthen the impact of NICE recommendations on sectors beyond the NHS and that work on the cost-effectiveness of public health interventions beyond clinical medicine be strengthened. At present, while economic modelling is well developed in clinical areas, particularly for pharmaceutical interventions, both methods and outcomes need further work in public health economics. A new funding stream for public health research in the UK (Milne and Law, 2009), a burgeoning of work on the costs and benefits of interventions with children, complex interventions and health promotion (for example, Rush et al., 2004; Roberts et al., 2008; Shiell et al., 2008; Shemilt et al., 2010; Bonin et al., 2011) the work of the Cochrane Campbell economics group, and the work of the those looking at the economics of education (e.g. Vignoles and Machin, 2005) mean that this field is likely to have a good deal to offer to those looking at the most (cost-) effective ways of reducing inequalities in child health.

In addition to needing further economic work on interventions, there is also a clear need for a register so that knowledge on public health interventions, can be shared (Waters et al., 2007). However, also needed, as Hawe (2011) points out, are the stories which researchers do not tell about unexplained outcomes, the unpublished findings which do not 'fit' and the research and the sense making across the whole piece. As she recommends, we need scholarship as well as research.

Legislation: breastfeeding

Scotland was the first country to make breastfeeding a legal right through legislation, although breastfeeding rates in the UK remain much lower than those in Scandinavia, which stand at around 98%.

Breastfeeding etc. (Scotland) Act 2005

The Bill for this Act of the Scottish Parliament was passed on 18th November 2004 and received Royal Assent on 18th January 2005.

An Act of the Scottish Parliament to make it an offence to prevent or stop a person in charge of a child who is otherwise permitted to be in a public place or licensed premises from feeding milk to that child in that place or on those premises; to make provision in relation to the promotion of breastfeeding; and for connected purposes.

www.legislation.gov.uk/asp/2005/1/introduction

Legislation: smoking

Smoking is a major threat to health, with a steep social class gradient in exposure of non-smokers, including children, both to tobacco, and tobacco use.

On July 1st 2007, England introduced a new law to make virtually all enclosed public places and workplaces in England smoke free. A longitudinal qualitative study (Hargreaves et al., 2010) identified reduced smoking in public places, and decreased reported consumption at one year post-legislation. The dominant pattern of reduced consumption was attributed primarily to constraints imposed by the legislation. Smoking behaviour was, however, strongly influenced by social networks, indicating that, while individuals had the power to act, any changes they made were largely shaped by social structural factors. The findings support the need for a comprehensive tobacco control strategy. Wakefield et al. (2000:333), in their study of 14- to 17-year-olds in 202 schools in the US, found that significantly associated with stage of smoking uptake were smoking restrictions in public places at home and at school. This suggests that smoking bans may reduce teenage smoking.

Fluoridation

Fluoridation in drinking water

A controlled trial of fluoridation in drinking water (Carmichael et al., 1989) was carried out in 1987 in the north east of England. The experimental group consisted of 457 children living in an area of drinking water fluoridation, and the control group of 370 children living in an area with no fluoridation. Both groups contained a wide socioeconomic range. Evaluation involved a dental examination and comparison with earlier studies. It was concluded that fluoridation led to reduced dental caries, mainly among children from more disadvantaged backgrounds, where the highest levels of caries had been found in earlier studies.

The single study described in the box above suggested that fluoridation could be a very attractive proposition, with real potential in reducing inequalities in health given the uneven distribution of dental caries in young children. However, things are not quite so straightforward.

In 1999, the Centre for Reviews and Dissemination (CRD) was commissioned to conduct a systematic review of the efficacy and safety of the fluoridation of drinking water to inform a policy decision-making process linked to legislation. It found that although a large number of studies had been conducted over the previous 50 years, there was a lack of reliable, good-quality evidence in the fluoridation literature worldwide. The available evidence suggested that water fluoridation reduces caries prevalence but it was unclear by how much since results of individual studies ranged from a substantial reduction to a slight increase. The research evidence was of insufficient quality to allow confident statements about potential harms other than mottling of the teeth, or about impact on inequalities. The evidence on benefits and harms, the authors suggested, needed to be considered along with the ethical, environmental, ecological, cost and legal issues that surround any decisions about water fluoridation (McDonagh et al., 2000). Wilson and Sheldon (2006:329), referring to the CRD review describe the way in which this was a relatively rare example of an explicit policy commitment to follow the findings of a review. Although the findings of such reviews may not be carried through if they contradict prior beliefs and policy intent, systematic reviews, with their comprehensive assessments of the evidence, are well-suited to putting controversial issues into the public domain, where they can be accessed by decision makers in other jurisdictions.

In November 2003, the House of Commons voted in favour of an amendment to the Water Bill. Under the amendment, water fluoridation takes place if a water company is asked to do so by a Strategic Health Authority, but only after public consultation at the local level has shown sufficient support for it. This debate exemplifies the point made by Mackenbach (2011) that a democratic mandate is needed to make large-scale policy changes.

Employment

A central plank of current government policy to reduce inequality is through work. This book is not the place for a full discussion of these initiatives, but there are substantial implications for child mental health of potential discontinuities in care if parental employment is not closely tied to good-quality, stable childcare. Many parents in work do not earn the minimum wage. *Closing the gap* (CSDH, 2008) suggests that the unequal distribution of health requires a strong public sector that is committed, capable and adequately financed. Part of this public sector is the workforce providing care to children and their families. The low pay and variable quality and standards for education and training of this workforce, together with the low status of those caring for children in the early years and those supporting families experiencing particular difficulties, are matters which require attention.

Policy implications of health inequalities research: dilemmas of advocacy

> 'You sometimes feel as if you're serenading outside a window, trying to get them to open it, singing "let me in." Sometimes you want to throw a brick in with a message tied to it. But there's no point in chanting from the outside. You really need to get inside the house, and how do you do that? ... You always think there are simple solutions. But in fact, it's very hard work.' (Respondent, R&D Team, 2000:48)

As Jessop (2006:297) points out, what is needed if health inequalities are to be significantly addressed are both technical fixes and then the political will to do something. While it is easy to point to failures of political will, unless we know what to do, political urgency may simply be translated into meetings, monitoring and bureaucracy. To that extent, the body of work which has been done over the last 20 years, and current research funding initiatives to evaluate what happens when these are turned into interventions, provide a bedrock for effective action.

Although Gunning-Schepers and Gepkens (1996: 235) pointed out that we could not count on health inequalities being high on the policy agenda for long, it has turned out that advocacy and lobbying have, in fact, maintained inequalities in health as a priority. Although policy influence and effective policy advocacy frequently depend on timing, most of the problems relating to inequalities are unlikely to disappear so quickly that evidence cannot be saved for a later opportunity. Changes to smoking legislation in Australia were dependent in part on the steady accumulation over time of good evidence which could be put to use when an opportunity arose, and researchers with a grasp of evidence-informed advocacy (Chapman, 2004). Epidemiologists working on injury and obesity have combined good science and powerful alliances.

Ian Roberts at the London School of Hygiene and Tropical Medicine, who is a trialist and a scientist, offers a perspective on advocacy:

> According to the dissident North American writer Noam Chomsky, the responsibility of academics is to speak the truth and to expose lies. Chomsky recognised that academics are a privileged minority 'with the leisure, facilities and training to seek the truth hidden behind the veil of distortion and misrepresentation, ideology and class interests through which the events of current history are presented to us.' More than any other discipline, public health provides an opportunity to take up Chomsky's challenge. (www.lshtm.ac.uk/prospectus/profiles/roberts.html)

Although different researchers will draw the science/advocacy/implementation line at different points, an increasing emphasis on impact may provide new perspectives on Max Weber's distinction between science as a vocation and politics as a vocation.

Recently on the research side, the two major reports (CSDH, 2008; Marmot, 2010), and on the policy side, the reports by Frank Field and Graham Allen (Field, 2010; Allen, 2011) have focused on what might be done. The Acheson report made clear that: 'without a shift of resources to the less well off, both in and out of work, little will be accomplished in terms of a reduction of health inequalities by addressing particular "downstream influences"' (Acheson, 1998:33). But those who seek to tackle inequalities in child health have found that evidence, however robust and comprehensive, does not translate seamlessly or automatically into policy, and that a good deal of policy is made in the absence of adequate evidence (Macintyre, 2011).

For policy change, political will is required, but so is political conviction. This presents a dilemma for policy advocacy. If the advocacy is conducted by a group of affected or concerned citizens – parents, patients, children – their argument depends on both the evidence at their disposal and their persistence and articulacy in using it. If evidence is being presented by researchers, they may be constrained from presenting it too vigorously lest they be dismissed as partisan and unscientific. On the other hand if they take no stand at all on evidence which calls into question what is currently not being done, or what is being harmfully done, they may appear to give scientific legitimacy to bad policies. It is a dilemma which potentially faces every researcher who hopes that policy will be shaped around the evidence, rather than the evidence tailored to fit the policy.

And finally...

The record of using evidence, in the widest possible sense, to inform and fuel policy and to ensure that the potential benefits for children are produced, enjoyed and sustained, gives grounds for optimism. Success is not easy, but it is possible, even by individual action. I had wanted to end the book with a positive example. The one I have chosen in the box that follows (from a website which promotes breastfeeding) is experience- rather than evidence-based, but it provides a parable on an example of the possibilities of individual action in starting to promote cultural change. I hope it will make readers smile.

Feel-good story

A number of years back I was in a restaurant as a party of four men for a business lunch, a couple of tables along there were a couple of mothers discreetly feeding while dining and a man on another table complained to the waiter. The waiter started asking the mothers to stop so I stood and called to the waiter that we would be leaving if he continued, he did continue. In a louder voice I asked for others to stand and support the mothers and about a dozen others also stood. The manager came out from somewhere, spoke to the waiter then the man who had complained and politely told him the women were welcome to feed if they wished and if he still objected he was welcome to leave after settling his bill, he rushed his meal and left. I told the manager to put the cost of the women's meals on my account; he promptly said he would not be charging them. When the women finished they packed their buggies and left, a few minutes later one returned, came over to our table and gave me a thank you card, we got into conversation and she said the two of them treated themselves to lunch out while they could as they had just heard that the company they worked for had gone into liquidation and lost their jobs and company's maternity pay. The result was one of the other guys in my party gave them both a job setting up and running a creche at his company and I became a godfather to both their babies. The restaurant set up a Kiddies area with more suitable seating for toddlers and feeding mothers and got more customers into the bargain.

www.007b.com/public-breastfeeding-europe.php

Key messages

For everyone
- Improving the prospects of children and young people is an investment rather than an expense.
- The investment required to eliminate child poverty is relatively small, amounting to 0.48% of GNP in the UK (UNICEF, 2000 in Spencer, 2000)
- Adequate income, affordable childcare, adult employment opportunities, an inclusive education system and accessible health, leisure and transport facilities are essential for the prevention and eradication of inequalities in child health.
- The Child Poverty Act 2010 legally binds the government to create a strategy to eradicate child poverty by 2020.
- A secure family income is one of the most important elements in enabling children to be healthy, to gain a good education, to live in a safe environment and to make choices about their future.

For the government
- A minimum income standard is needed to maintain good health and the well-being of children; parents need to earn a living wage.
- For sustainable impact of initiatives of known effectiveness, long-term mainstream funding is needed.

- Tax increases are the single most effective intervention to reduce demand for tobacco.
- Investment is needed in the childcare workforce.

For those involved in commissioning services
- Improving the health of children and young people needs to be a key R&D priority, with an emphasis on the 'D' for development.
- The costs of monitoring a service can be set against the costs of running an ineffective service.

References

Aaro, L., Hauknes, A. and Berglund, E. (1981) 'Smoking among Norwegian school children 1975 – 1980: the influence of the social environment', *Scandinavian Journal of Psychology*, 22, pp 297–309.

Acheson, D. (1998*) Independent inquiry into inequalities in health*, ('Acheson report'), London: The Stationery Office.

Action on Access (2010) *The Frank Buttle Trust quality mark: a practice guide*, www. actiononaccess.org/resources/files/resources__Best Practice Guide – Final Version.pdf.

Aicken, C., Arai, L., Roberts, H. (2008) *Schemes to promote healthy weight among obese and overweight children in England*, London: EPPI-Centre, Social Science Research Unit, Institute of Education, University of London.

Aicken, C., Roberts, H., Arai, L. (2010) 'Mapping service activity: the example of childhood obesity schemes in England', *BMC Public Health*, June 4, 10(1), p 310.

Alderson, P. and Morrow, V. (2011) *The ethics of research with children and young people: a practical handbook*, London: Sage Publications.

Allen, G. (2011) *Early intervention: the next steps,* London: HM Government.

Allen, M. and Burrell, N. (1996) 'Comparing the impact of homosexual and heterosexual parents on children: meta-analysis of existing research', *Journal of Homosexuality*, 32, pp 19–35.

Ampofo-Boateng, K. and Thomson, J.A. (1989) 'Child pedestrian accidents: a case for preventive medicine', *Health Education Research*, 5, pp 265–74.

Andrews, E. (2009) *Disabled Children's Access to Childcare (DCATCH) pilot activity*, London: DCSF.

Arai, L. (2009) *Teenage pregnancy: the making and unmaking of a problem*, Bristol: Policy Press.

Arblaster, L., Lambert, M., Entwistle, V., Forster, M., Fullerton, D., Sheldon, T. and Watt, I. (1996) 'A systematic review of the effectiveness of health service interventions aimed at reducing inequalities in health', *Journal of Health Services Research and Policy*, 1(2), pp 93–103.

Arblaster, L., Entwhistle, V., Fullerton, D., Forster, M., Lambert, M. and Sheldon, T.A. (1997) *A review of the effectiveness of health promotion intervention aimed at reducing inequalities in health: CRD report,* York: NHS Centre for Reviews and Dissemination, University of York.

Armstrong, R., Waters, E., Dobbins, M., Lavis, J.N., Petticrew, M. and Christensen, R. (2011) 'Knowledge translation strategies for facilitating evidence-informed public health decision making among managers and policy-makers (Protocol)', *Cochrane Database of Systematic Reviews*, Issue 6, DOI: 10.1002/14651858. CD009181.

Ashton-Key, M. and Jorge, E. (2003) 'Does providing social services with information and advice on immunisation status of "looked after children" improve uptake?', *Archives of Disease in Childhood,* 88, pp 299-301.

Barker, D.J.P. (1994) *Mothers, babies and disease in later life*, London: British Medical Journal Publications.

Barker, E.D., Oliver, B.R., Viding, E., Salekin, R.T. and Maughan, B. (2011) 'The impact of prenatal maternal risk, fearless temperament and early parenting on adolescent callous-unemotional traits: a 14-year longitudinal investigation', *Journal of Child Psychology and Psychiatry*, 52(8), pp 878–88.

Barlow, J., Smailagic, N., Ferriter, M., Bennett, C. and Jones, H. (2010) 'Group-based parent-training programmes for improving emotional and behavioural adjustment in children from birth to three years old', *Cochrane Database of Systematic Reviews*, Issue 3, DOI: 10.1002/14651858.CD003680.pub2

Barlow, J., Smailagic, N., Bennett, C., Huband, N., Jones, H. and Coren, E. (2011) 'Individual and group based parenting programmes for improving psychosocial outcomes for teenage parents and their children', Cochrane Database of Systematic Reviews, Issue 3. Art. No.: CD002964. DOI: 10.1002/14651858. CD002964.pub2

Barn, R., Andrew, L. and Mantovani, N. (2005) *The experiences of young care leavers from different ethnic groups*, York: Joseph Rowntree Foundation.

Barnard, M.A. (2003) 'Between a rock and a hard place: the role of relatives in protecting children from the effects of parental drug problems', *Child and Family Social Work*, 8(4), pp 291–9.

Barnard, M.A. (2005a) 'Discomforting research: colliding moralities and looking for "truth" in a study of parental drug problems', *Sociology of Health and Illness*, 27(1), pp 1-19.

Barnard, M.A. (2005b) *Drugs in the family: the impact on parents and siblings*, York: Joseph Rowntree Foundation.

Barnard, M.A. and McKeganey, N.P. (2004) 'The impact of parental problem drug use on children: what is the problem and what is being done to help?' *Addiction*, 99(5), pp 552–9.

Barnardo's (2008-09) *Marlborough Road Partnership*, www.barnardos.org.uk/marlboroughroad.htm

Barnardo's R&D [Research and Development] Team (2000) *Making connections: linking research and practice*, Barkingside: Barnardo's.

Barnett, W.S. (1993) 'Cost benefit analysis,' in L.J. Schweinhart, H.V. Barnes and D.P. Weikart (eds) *The High/Scope Perry Preschool Study through age 27*, Ypsilanti: High/Scope Educational Research Foundation.

Barnsdale, L. and Walker, M. (2007) *Examining the use and impact of family group conferences*, Edinburgh: Scottish Government, www.scotland.gov.uk/Publications/2007/03/26093721/0

Bartington, S., Griffiths, L., Tate, A.R., Dezateux, C. and the Millennium Cohort Study Child Health Group (2006) 'Are breastfeeding rates higher among mothers delivering in baby friendly accredited maternity units in the UK?' *International Journal of Epidemiology* 35(5): 1178-1186. doi: 10.1093/ije/dyl155 First published online: 22 August.

Baughcum A.E., Burklow K.A., Deeks C.M., Powers S.W., Whitaker R.C. (1998) 'Maternal feeding practices and childhood obesity: a focus group study of low-income mothers', Archives of *Pediatrics & Adolescent Medicine*, 152, pp 1010–14.

Beecham, J., Greco V., Sloper, P. and Webb, R. (2007) 'The costs of key worker support for disabled children and their families', *Child: Care, Health and Development*, 33(5), pp 611–18.

Bell, C. and Newby, H. (1977) *Doing sociological research*, London: Allen and Unwin.

Bell, C. and Roberts, H. (1984) *Social researching: politics, problems, practice*, London: Routledge and Kegan Paul.

Belsky, J., Melhuish, E., Barnes, J., Leyland, A.H., Romaniuk, H. and the National Evaluation of Sure Start Research Team (2006) 'Effects of Sure Start local programmes on children and families: early findings from a quasi-experimental, cross sectional study', *British Medical Journal*, 332 p 1476 doi: 10.1136/British Medical Journal.38853.451748.2F

Bennett, E. (2010) *Counting the costs: the financial realities for families with disabled children*, London: Contact a Family, www.cafamily.org.uk/pdfs/CountingtheCosts2010.pdf

Benzeval, M., Der, G., Ellaway, A., Hunt, K., Sweeting, H., West, P. and Macintyre, S. (2009) 'Cohort profile: West of Scotland 20-07 study: health in the community', *International Journal of Epidemiology*, 38, pp 1215-23.

Beresford, B. and Clarke, S. (2010) *Improving the wellbeing of disabled children and young people through improving access to positive and inclusive activities*, York: Social Policy Research Unit, University of York.

Beresford, B., Sloper, P., Baldwin S. and Newman, T. (1996) *What works for families with a disabled child?* Barkingside: Barnardo's.

Berridge, D., Henry, L., Jackson, S. and Turney, D. (2009) *Looked after and learning: evaluation of the Virtual School Head pilot,* London: Department for Children, Schools and Families.

Berrueta-Clement, J.R., Schweinhart, L.J., Barnett, W.S., Epstein, A.S. and Weikart, D.P. (1984) *Changed lives: the effects of the Perry Pre-school Program on youths through age 19.* Ypsilanti: High/Scope Press.

Biehal, N., Clayden, J., Stein, M. and Wade, J. (1995) *Moving on: young people and leaving care schemes,* Barkingside: Barnardo's.

Bird, W. (2007) *Natural thinking,* RSPB, www.rspb.org.uk/Images/naturalthinking_tcm9-161856.pdf.

Birkett, D. (2011) The children's manifesto, *Guardian*, 3 May, www.guardian.co.uk/education/2011/may/03/school-i-would-like-childrens-manifesto.

Black, D. (1980) see Working Group on Inequalities in Health (1980).

Black, R.E., Cousens, S., Johnson, H.L. et al. (2010) 'Global, regional, and national causes of child mortality in 2008: a systematic analysis', *Lancet,* 375, pp 1969–87.

Blackburn, C., Read, J. and Spencer, N. (2007) 'Can we count them? Scoping data sources on disabled children and their households in the UK', *Child: Care, Health and Development,* 33(3), pp 291–5.

Bond, L. and Butler, H. (2009) 'The Gatehouse Project: a multi-level integrated approach to promoting wellbeing in schools', in A. Killoran and M. Kelly (eds) *Evidence-based public health: effectiveness and efficiency,* Oxford: Oxford University Press, pp 250-69.

Bonell, C., Fletcher, A. and McCambridge, J. (2007) 'Improving school ethos may reduce substance misuse and teenage pregnancy', *British Medical Journal,* 334(7594), pp 614–6.

Bonin, E., Stevens, M., Beecham, J., Byford, S. and Parsonage, M. (2011) 'Costs and longer-term savings of parenting programmes for the prevention of persistent conduct disorder: a modelling study', www.biomedcentral.com/1471-2458/11/803.

Boreham, R. and Blenkinsop, S. (eds) (2004) *Drug use, smoking and drinking among young people in England in 2003,* London: Stationery Office.

Boruch, R.F. and Riecken, H.W. (eds) (1975) *Experimental testing of public policy,* Boulder, CO: Westview Press.

Bostock, L. (1998) ' "It's Catch-22 all the time': mothers' experiences of caring on low income in the 1990s" ', [unpublished PhD thesis], Lancaster: Lancaster University.

Botting, B., Rosato, M. and Wood, R. (1998) 'Teenage mothers and the health of their children', *Population Trends,* 93 (Autumn), pp 19–28.

Broad, B., Hayes, R. and Rushforth, C. (2001) *Kith and kin: kinship care for vulnerable young people,* York: Joseph Rowntree Foundation.

Brown, T. and Summerbell, C.D. (2009) 'Systematic review of school-based interventions that focus on changing dietary intake and physical activity levels to prevent childhood obesity: an update to the obesity guidance produced by the National Institute for Health and Clinical Excellence', *Obesity Reviews,* 10(1), pp 110–141.

Buchanan, A. and Ritchie, C. (2004) *What works for troubled children?* Barkingside: Barnardo's, www.barnardos.org.uk/what_works_for_troubled_children__-_summary_1_.pdf

Bunker, J. (2001) *Medicine matters after all: measuring the benefits of medical care, a healthy lifestyle, and a just social environment,* London: The Nuffield Trust.

Bunn, F., Collier T., Frost, C., Ker, K., Steinbach, R., Roberts, I. and Wentz, R. (2003) 'Area-wide traffic calming for preventing traffic related injuries (Cochrane Review)', *Cochrane Database of Systematic Reviews,* Issue 1, DOI: 10.1002/14651858.CD003110.

Butland, B., Jebb, S., Kopelman, P., McPherson., K, Thomas, S. and Mardell, J. (2007) *Foresight: tackling obesities: future choices – project report. 2007,* London: Department of Innovation, Universities and Skills.

Butler, H., Bowes, G., Drew, S., Glover, S., Godfrey, C., Patton, G., Trafford, L. and Bond, L. (2010) 'Harnessing complexity: taking advantage of context and relationships in dissemination of school-based interventions', *Health Promotion Practice,* 11, pp 259–67.

Bynner, J. and Joshi, H. (2002) 'Equality and opportunity in education: evidence from the 1958 and 1970 birth cohort studies', *Oxford Review of Education*, 28(4), pp 405–25.

Caird, J., Kavanagh, J., Oliver, K., Oliver, S., O'Mara, A., Stansfield, C. and Thomas, J. (2011) *Childhood obesity and educational attainment: a systematic review,* London: EPPI-Centre, Social Science Research Unit, Institute of Education, University of London.

Calouste Gulbenkian Foundation (1995) *Children and violence*, London: Calouste Gulbenkian.

Cameron, D. (2009) *Hugo Young memorial lecture,* November 10, 2009, www.conservatives.com/News/Speeches/2009/11/David_Cameron_The_Big_Society.aspx.

CAPT and Roberts, H. (1993) *A safe school is no accident*, London: Child Accident Prevention Trust.

Carless, A. (1921) 'Medical report', in *Dr. Barnardo's Homes annual report*, Barkingside: Barnardo's, pp 23–8.

Carmichael, C.L., Rugg-Gunn, A.J. and Ferrell R.S. (1989) 'The relationship between fluoridation, social class and caries experience in 5 year old children in Newcastle and Northumberland in 1987', *British Dental Journal*, 167, pp 57–61.

Carr-Hill, R.A., Rugg-Gunn, A.J. and Ferrell, R.S. (1994) *A formula for distributing NHS revenues based on small area use*, Occasional Paper, York: Centre for Health Economics, University of York.

Chamba, R., Ahmad, W., Hirst, D., Lawton D. and Beresford, B. (1999) *On the edge: minority ethnic families caring for a severely disabled child*, Bristol: The Policy Press for the Joseph Rowntree Foundation, York.

Chapman, S. (2004) 'Advocacy for public health: a primer', *Journal of Epidemiology and Community Health,* 58, pp 361–5.

Cheung, Y. and Heath, A. (1994) 'After care: the education and occupation of adults who have been in care', *Oxford Review of Education*, 20(3), pp 361–74.

ChildLine (2008) *Children talking to ChildLine about bullying,* www.nspcc.org.uk/inform/publications/casenotes/children_talking_to_childline_about_bullying_wda61701.html

ChildLine (2011) *Looked after children talking to ChildLine*, ChildLine Casenotes, London: NSPCC, www.nspcc.org.uk/Inform/publications/casenotes/clcasenoteslookedafterchildren_wdf80622.pdf

Children's Rights Director for England (2007) *Children on care standards: children's views on national minimum standards for children's social care: a report by the Children's Rights Director for England*, London: OFSTED.

Cleaver, H. and Freeman, P. (1995) *Parental perspectives in cases of suspected child abuse*, London: HMSO.

Cleaver, H., Nicholson, D., Tarr, S. and Cleaver, D. (2007) *Child protection, domestic violence and parental substance misuse,* London: Jessica Kingsley.

Cockman, P., Dawson, L., Mathur, R. and Hull, S. (2011) 'Improving MMR vaccination rates: herd immunity is a realistic goal', *British Medical Journal*, 343:bmj.d5703.

Cole-Hamilton, I. (2002) *Something good and fun: children's and parents' views on play and out-of-school provision*, London: Children's Play Council.

Cole-Hamilton, I. and Lang, T. (1986) *Tightening belts: a report of the impact of poverty on food*, London: London Food Commission.

Coleman, J.M. (2005) 'In spite of informed consent: limitations of human research ethics processes when a clinical drug trial is abruptly terminated', [unpublished PhD thesis], Victoria, Australia: School of Public Health, La Trobe University.

Collison, D., Dey, C., Hannah, G. and Stevenson, L. (2007) 'Income inequality and child mortality in wealthy nations', *Journal of Public Health*, 29(2), pp 114–17, doi. 10.1093/PUBMED/FDM009.

Conde-Agudelo, A., Belizán, J.M. and Diaz-Rossello, J. (2011) 'Kangaroo mother care to reduce morbidity and mortality in low birthweight infants', *Cochrane Database of Systematic Reviews*, Issue 3, DOI: 10.1002/14651858.CD002771.pub2.

Connell, J.P. and Kubisch, A.C. (1998) 'Applying a theory of change approach to the evaluation of comprehensive community initiatives: progress, prospects, and problems', in K. Fulbright-Anderson, A.C. Kubisch and J.P. Connell (eds) *New approaches to evaluating community initiatives: volume 2 – theory, measurement, and analysis*, Washington, DC: The Aspen Institute.

Connelly, G., Forest, J. and Furnival, J. (2008) *The educational attainment of looked after children: local authority pilot projects final research report*, Edinburgh: The Scottish Government.

Craig, P., Dieppe, P., Macintyre, S., Michie, S., Nazareth, I. and Petticrew, M. (2008) 'Developing and evaluating complex interventions: the new Medical Research Council guidance', *British Medical Journal*, 337, pp a1655.

CRD (2000) 'Promoting the initiation of breastfeeding', *Effective Healthcare Bulletin*, 6(2), www.york.ac.uk/inst/crd/EHC/ehc62.pdf.

CSDH (2008) *Closing the gap in a generation: health equity through action on the social determinants of health*, Geneva: WHO.

CYPU (2002) *Have your say consultation*, London: Children and Young People's Unit.

Davey Smith, G., Bartley, M. and Blane, D. (1990) 'The Black report on socio-economic inequalities in health ten years on', *British Medical Journal*, 301, pp 373–77.

Davies, C. and Ward, H. (2011) *Safeguarding children across services: messages from research*, London: Jessica Kingsley.

Davis, R. and Pless, B. (2001) 'British Medical Journal bans "accidents"', *British Medical Journal*, 322, p 1320.

DCSF Schools Analysis and Research Division (2009) *Deprivation and education: the evidence on pupils in England, Foundation Stage to Key Stage 4*. London: DCSF www.education.gov.uk/publications/eOrderingDownload/DCSF-RTP-09-01.pdf.

Dearlove, J. (1999) *Support needs of women on low income caring for children*, Coventry: University of Warwick.

Department for Education (2011) *16- to 18-year-olds not in education, employment or training* (NEET) www.education.gov.uk/16to19/participation/neet/a0064101/16-to-18-year-olds-not-in-education-employment-or-training-neet.

Department for Transport (2000a) *New directions in speed management: a review of policy*, London: Department for Transport. http://people.pwf.cam.ac.uk/jc235/Speed%20Limits/Annex%20toSpeed%20Management%20.pdf.

Department for Transport (2000b) *Report on the Gloucester Safer City Project*, London: Department for Transport.

Department of Health (1995) *Child protection: messages from research*, London: HMSO.

Department of Health (2000) *Protecting children, supporting parents: a consultation document of the physical punishment of children*, London: DoH. http://dera.ioe.ac.uk/1780/1/dh_4054848.pdf.

Department of Health (2008) *Mortality target monitoring (infant mortality, inequalities) update to include data for 2008*, www.dh.gov.uk/en/Publicationsandstatistics/Publications/PublicationsStatistics/DH_109161.

Department of Health (2009) *Healthy lives, brighter futures*, London: Department of Health, www.dh.gov.uk/en/Publicationsandstatistics/Publications/PublicationsPolicyAndGuidance/DH_094400.

Department of Health (2010) *Equity and excellence: Liberating the NHS*, London: Department of Health.

Department of Health (nd) *The Family Nurse Partnership Programme*, www.dh.gov.uk/en/Publicationsandstatistics/Publications/PublicationsPolicyAndGuidance/DH_118530.

Dex, S. and Joshi, H. (2005) *Children of the 21st century: From birth to nine months*, Bristol: The Policy Press.

DiGuiseppi, C. and Higgins, J.P.T. (2001) 'Interventions for promoting smoke alarm ownership and function' *Cochrane Database of Systematic Reviews 2001*, (2):CD002246.

DiGuiseppi, C., Roberts, I., Wade, A., Sculpher, M., Edwards, P., Godward, C., Pan, H. and Slater, S. (2002) 'Incidence of fires and related injuries after giving out free smoke alarms: cluster randomised controlled trial', *British Medical Journal*, 325(7371) p 995.

Dixon, J. and Stein, M. (2002) *A study of throughcare and aftercare services in Scotland*. Scotland's Children, Research Findings No. 3, Edinburgh: Scottish Executive.

Douglas, J.W.B. (1986) *The home and the school*, London: MacGibbon and Kee.

Doyle, A. (1875) *Pauper children (Canada), Return to an Order of the Honourable, The House of Commons dated 8 February*, London: HMSO.

DTI (1995) *Home accident surveillance system annual report 1995*, London: DTI.

DuBois, D.L., Holloway, B.E., Valentine, J.C. and Cooper, H. (2002) 'Effectiveness of mentoring programs for youth: a meta-analytic review', *American Journal of Community Psychology*, 30, pp 157–97.

Dunne, M., Dyson, A., Gallannaugh, F., Humphreys, S., Muijs, D. and Sebba, J. (2007) *Effective teaching and learning for pupils in low attaining groups*, Research report DCSF-RR011, London: DCSF.

Duperrex, O., Roberts, I.G. and Bunn, F. (2002a) 'Safety education of pedestrians for injury prevention', *Cochrane Database of Systematic Reviews 2002*, Issue 2, DOI: 10.1002/14651858.CD001531.

Duperrex, O., Bunn, F. and Roberts, I. (2002b) 'Safety education of pedestrians for injury prevention', *British Medical Journal*, 324(7346), pp 1129–31.

Dyson, A. and Gallannaugh, F. (2008) 'Disproportionality in special needs education in England', *The Journal of Special Education*, 42(1), 36–46.

Dyson, A., Gunter, H., Hall, D., Raffo, C., Jones, L. and Kalambouka, A. (2010) 'What is to be done? Implications for policy makers', in C. Raffo, D. Dyson, H.M. Gunter, D. Hall, L. Jones and A. Kalambouka (eds) *Education and poverty in affluent countries*, London: Routledge.

Eckenrode, J., Campa, M., Luckey, D.W., Henderson C.R. Jr., Cole, R., Kitzman, H., Anson, E., Sidora-Arcoleo, K., Powers, J. and Olds, D.L. (2010) 'Long-term effects of prenatal and infancy nurse home visitation on the life course of youths: 19-year follow-up of a randomized trial', *Archives of Pediatrics and Adolescent Medicine,* 164(1), pp 9–15.

Edholm, F., Roberts H. and Sayer, J. (1983) *Vietnamese refugees in Britain*, London: Commission for Racial Equality.

Edwards, P., Roberts, I., Green, J. and Lutchmun, S. (2006) 'Deaths from injury in children and employment status in family: analysis of trends in class specific death rates', *British Medical Journal*, 333(7559), p 119, www.bmj.com/content/333/7559/119

Edwards, B., Gray, M., Wise, S., Hayes, A., Katz, I., Muir, K. and Patulny, R. (2011) 'Early impacts of Communities for Children on children and families: findings from a quasi-experimental cohort study', *Journal of Epidemiology and Community Health,* 65, pp 909–14.

Eiser, J.R., Morgan, M., Gammage, P. and Gray, E. (1989) 'Adolescent smoking: attitudes, norms and parental influence', *British Journal of Psychology*, 28, pp 193–202.

Elliott, J. (2008) 'Fifty years of change in British society' in J. Elliott and R. Vaitilingam (eds) *Now we are 50: key findings from the National Child Development Study*. London: Centre for Longitudinal Studies, Institute of Education, University of London.

Elvik, R. (2001) 'Area-wide urban traffic calming schemes: a meta-analysis of safety effects', *Accident Analysis and Prevention*, 33(3), pp 327–36.

Farmer, E. and Owen, M. (1995) *Child protection practice: private risks and public remedies: decision making, intervention and outcome in child protection work,* London: HMSO.

Farran, D.C. (1990) 'Effects of intervention with disadvantaged and disabled children: a decade review', in S.J. Meisels and J.P. Shonkoff (eds) *Handbook of early childhood intervention*, Cambridge: Cambridge University Press.

Farrington, D.P. and Ttofi, M.M. (2010) 'School based programmes to reduce bullying and victimisation', *Campbell Collaboration* www.campbellcollaboration.org/news_/reduction_bullying_schools.php.

Ferri, E. (ed) (1993) *Life at 33: The fifth follow up of the National Child Development Survey*, London: National Children's Bureau and City University.

Field, F. (2010) *The foundation years: preventing poor children becoming poor adults,* London: HM Government.

Flenady,V., Middleton, P., Smith, G.C. and Duke,W. (2011) *Stillbirths: the way forward in high-income countries*, for The Lancet's Stillbirths Series steering committee.

Forrester, D. and Harwin, J. (2011) *Parents who misuse drugs and alcohol: effective interventions in social work and child protection*, London: John Wiley and Sons.

Gallagher, J.F. (1990) 'The family as a focus for intervention', in S.J. Meisels and J.P. Shonkoff (eds) *Handbook of early childhood intervention*, Cambridge: Cambridge University Press.

Garcia, J., France-Dawson, M.F. and Macfarlane, A. (1994) *Improving infant health*, London: HEA.

Garforth, S. and Garcia, J. (1989) 'Breastfeeding policies in practice: "No wonder they get confused" ', *Midwifery*, 5, pp 75–83.

Gibbs, L., Abebe, M. and Riggs, E. (2009) 'Working with minority groups in developed countries'. in E.Waters, J. Seidell, B. Swinburn and R. Uauy (eds) *Community-based childhood obesity prevention: Evidence, policy and practice*, Oxford: Wiley Blackwell Publishing.

Gilbert, R., Spatz,W.C., Browne, K., Fergusson, D.,Webb, E. and Janson, S. (2009a) 'Burden and consequences of child maltreatment in high-income countries', *Lancet,* 373(9657), pp 68–81.

Gilbert, R., Kemp, A. and Thoburn, J.(2009b) 'Recognising and responding to child maltreatment', *Lancet* 373(9658), pp 167–180.

Gilmore, H.C. (1950) 'Medical report', in *Dr. Barnardo's Homes Annual Report*, Barkingside: Barnardo's, pp 20 –21.

Glass, N. (1999) 'Sure Start: the development of an early intervention programme for young children in the United Kingdom', *Children and Society*, 13, pp 257–64.

Glasziou, P.,Vandenbroucke, J.P. and Chalmers, I. (2004) 'Assessing the quality of research', *British Medical Journal*, 328(7430), pp 39-41.

Golding. J., Fleming, P. and Parkes, S. (1992) 'Cot deaths and sleep position campaigns', *Lancet*, 339(8795), pp 748-9.

Goodman, R. (1997) 'Child mental health: who is responsible?', *British Medical Journal*, 314, pp 813 –17.

Gordon, L. (1988) *Heroes in their own lives: the politics and history of family violence*, London:Virago.

Graham, H. (1993a) *Hardship and health in women's lives*, Brighton: Harvester Wheatsheaf.

Graham, H. (1993b) *When life's a drag: women smoking and disadvantage*, London: HMSO.

Graham, H. and Kelly, M. (2004) *Health inequalities: concepts, frameworks and policy: briefing paper*, London: Health Development Agency.

Gray, J.A.M. (1997) *Evidence-based health care: how to make health policy and management decisions*, New York and London: Churchill Livingstone.

Gray,J.A.M. (2000) 'Promoting an evaluative culture', *Public Health Forum,* 3(2), p. 8.

Gray, R. and McCormick, M. (2009) 'Socioeconomic inequalities in survival in neonates', *British Medical Journal,* 339:bmj.b5041 .

Gray, R., Hollowell, J., Brocklehurst, P., Graham, H. and Kurinczuk, J. (2009) *Health inequalities infant mortality target: technical background*, Oxford: Perinatal Epidemiology Unit.

Green, H., McGinnity, Á., Meltzer, H., Ford, T. and Goodman, R. (2005) *Mental health of children and young people in Great Britain, 2004*, HMSO/Palgrave Macmillan, www.esds.ac.uk/doc/5269/mrdoc/pdf/5269technicalreport.pdf.

Green, J. (2001) 'Reply to Davis and Pless', *British Medical Journal*, www.bmj.com/content/322/7298/1320.full/reply#bmj_el_16290

Grossman, J.B. and Rhodes, J.E. (2002) 'The test of time: predictors and effects of duration in youth mentoring programs', *American Journal of Community Psychology*, 30, pp 199–206.

Guardian (1994) 'Editorial', July 28.

Gunning-Schepers, L.J. and Gepkens, A. (1996) 'Reviews of interventions to reduce social inequalities in health: research and policy implications', *Health Education Journal*, 55, pp 226–38.

Gutman, L.M. and Feinstein, L. (2008) *Children's well-being in primary school: pupil and school effects*, www.learningbenefits.net/Publications/ResRepIntros/ResRep25intro.htm

Gutman, L.M., Brown, J. and Akerman, R. (2010) *Nurturing parenting capability: why do parents parent the way they do? Extension report on predictors of parenting at five years*, www.learningbenefits.net/Publications/DiscussionPapers/parenting_extension_11-08_FINAL2.pdf.

Haddon, W., Suchman, E. and Klein, D. (eds) (1964) *Accident research: methods and approaches*, New York: Evanston and London: Harper and Row.

Hagger-Johnson, G., Batty, G.D., Deary, I.J. and von Stumm, S. (2011) 'Childhood socioeconomic status and adult health: comparative formative and reflective models in the Aberdeen Children of the 1950s Study (prospective cohort study)', *Journal of Epidemiology and Community Health*, 65(11), pp 1024–9.

Halladay, M. and Bero, L. (2000) 'Implementing evidence-based practice in health care', *Public Money and Management*, 20, pp 43–50.

Hammond, C. and Feinstein, L. (2006) *Are those who flourished at school healthier adults? What role for adult education?* London: Centre for Research on the Wider Benefits of Learning, Institute of Education.

Happer, H., McCreadie, J. and Aldgate, J. (2006) *Celebrating success: what helps looked after children succeed?* Edinburgh: The Scottish Government.

Hargreaves, K., Amos, A., Highet, G., Martin, C., Platt, S., Ritchie, D. and White, M. (2010) 'The social context of change in tobacco consumption following the introduction of "smokefree" England legislation: a qualitative, longitudinal study', *Social Science and Medicine*, 71(3), pp 459–466.

Harwin, J., Ryan, M., Tinnard, J. with Pokhrel, S., Alrouh, B., Matias, C. and Momenian-Schneider, S. (2011) *The Family Drug and Alcohol Court (FDAC) Evaluation Project: final report*, London: Brunel University, www.brunel.ac.uk/7067/FDAC/FDACEVALUATIONFINALREPORTMay2011.pdf.

Hauser-Cram, P. (1990) 'Designing meaningful evaluations of early intervention services', in S.J. Meisels and J.P. Shonkoff (eds.) *Handbook of early childhood intervention*, Cambridge: Cambridge University Press.

Hawe, P. (2011) 'The truth, but not the whole truth? Call for an amnesty on unreported results of public health interventions', *Journal of Epidemiology and Community Health*, Online First, published on October 14 as 10.1136/jech.2011.140350.

Hawe, P., Shiell, A. and Riley, T. (2009) 'Theorising interventions as events in systems', *American Journal of Community Psychology,* 43(3–4), pp 267–76.

Hawkes, D., Joshi, H. and Ward, K. (2004) *Unequal entry to motherhood and unequal start to life: evidence from the first survey of the UK Millennium Cohort,* CLS Cohort Studies Working Paper No.6, London: Centre for Longitudinal Studies, Institute of Education.

HEC (1987) *The health divide: inequalities in health in the 1980s,* London: Health Education Council

Hill, C.M., Mather, M. and Goddard, J. (2003) 'Cross sectional survey of meningococcal C immunisation in children looked after by local authorities and those living at home', *British Medical Journal*, 326(7385), pp 364–5.

Hill, G. (2002) '(letter) Smoke alarms', 2 November www.bmj.com/content/325/7371/979.full/reply#bmj_el_26666.

Hillman, M., Adams, J.G.U. and Whitelegg, J. (1990) *One false move: a study of children's independent mobility*, London: Policy Studies Institute.

Hirsch, D. (2008) *What is needed to end child poverty in 2020?* York: Joseph Rowntree Foundation.

HM Treasury (2004a) *Child poverty review*, London: The Stationery Office.

HM Treasury (2004b) *Delivering stability: securing our future housing needs,* London: HM Treasury, http://webarchive.nationalarchives.gov.uk/+/www.hm-treasury. gov.uk/barker_review_of_housing_supply_recommendations.htm.

HM Treasury (2008) *Ending child poverty: everybody's business.* London: H M Treasury. www.hm-treasury.gov.uk/d/bud08_childpoverty_1310.pdf.

Hoddinott, P. and Pill, R. (2000) 'A qualitative study of women's views about how health professionals communicate about infant feeding', *Health Expectations*, 3(4), pp 224–33.

Hoddinott, P., Lee, A.J. and Pill, R. (2006) 'Effectiveness of a breastfeeding peer coaching intervention in rural Scotland', *Birth*, 33, pp 27–36.

Hollowell, J., Kurinczuk, J., Brocklehurst, P. and Gray, R. (2011) 'Social and ethnic inequalities in infant mortality: a perspective from the United Kingdom', *Seminars in Perinatology*, 5(4), pp 240–4.

Holtermann, S. (1995) *All Our futures: the impact of public expenditure and fiscal policies on Britain's children and young people*, Barkingside: Barnardo's.

Holy Bible, Authorised Version, Oxford: Oxford University Press, Book of Daniel, Chapter I, vv 10–16.

Horta, B. L., Bahl, R., Martines, J. C. and Victora, C. G. (2007) *Evidence on the long-term effects of breastfeeding: systematic reviews and meta-analyses,* Geneva: World Health Organization.

Howden-Chapman, P., Matheson, A., Crane, J., Viggers, H., Cunningham, M., Blakely, T., Cunningham, C., Woodward, A., Saville-Smith, K., O'Dea, D., Kennedy, M., Baker, M., Waipara, N., Chapman, R. and Davie, G. (2007) 'Effect of insulating houses on health inequality: cluster randomised study in the community', *British Medical Journal*, 334, p 460.

Howden-Chapman, P., Pierse, N. and Nicholls, S. (2008) 'Effects of improved home heating on asthma in community dwelling children: randomised controlled trial' *British Medical Journal*, 337:a1411, doi: 10.1136/bmj.a1411.

Howell, E.A., Herbert, P. Chatterjee, S., Kleinman, L.C. and Chassin, M.B. (2008) 'Black/white differences in very low birth weight neonatal mortality rates among New York City hospitals', *Pediatrics*, 121:e 407–15.

HSE and Molloy, B. (2011) *Annual report: Community Mothers Programme 2010*, www.lenus.ie/hse/bitstream/10147/136802/1/CommMothers2010.pdf.

Hugh-Jones, S. and Smith, P. (1999) 'Self-reports of short- and long-term effects of bullying on children who stammer', *British Journal of Educational Psychology*, 69, pp 141–58.

Hutson, S. (1997) *Supported housing: the experience of young care leavers*, Barkingside: Barnardo's.

Hyndeman, S.J. (1990) 'Housing dampness and health among British Bengalis in East London', *Social Science and Medicine*, 30, pp 131–41.

Illsley, R. (1967) 'The Sociological study of reproduction and its outcome', in S. A. Richardson and A.F. Guttmacher (eds) *Childbearing: its social and psychological aspects*, Baltimore, MD: Williams and Wilkins.

Information Centre (2006) *Drug use, smoking and drinking among young people in England 2004*, Leeds: The Information Centre.

Irwin, L.G., Siddiqi, A. and Hertzman, C. (2007) *Early child development: a powerful equalizer: final report of the Early Child Development Knowledge Network of the Commission on Social Determinants of Health*, Geneva: World Health Organization.

Jackson, S. and Sachdev, D. (2001) *Better education, better futures: research, practice and the views of young people in public care*, Barkingside: Barnardo's.

Jackson, S. and Thomas, N. (1999) *On the move again? What works in creating stability for looked after children*, Barkingside: Barnardo's.

Jackson, S., Ajayi, S. and Quigley, M. (2005) *Going to university from care: final report By Degrees Project*, London: Institute of Education.

Jensen, G.B. and Hampton, J. (2007) 'Early termination of drug trials: what are the ramifications for drug companies and drug safety monitoring boards?', *British Medical Journal*, 334, p 326.

Jessop, E.J. (2006) 'Another public health triumph', *Journal of Public Health*, 28(4), pp 297–8.

Johnson, Z., Howell, F. and Molloy, B. (1993) 'Community Mothers Programme: randomised controlled trial of non-professional intervention in parenting', *British Medical Journal*, 306, pp 1449–52.

Johnson, Z. Molloy, B., Scallan, E., Fitzpatrick, P., Rooney, B., Keegan, T. and Byrne, P. (2000) 'Community Mothers Programme: seven year follow-up of a randomised controlled trial of non-professional intervention in parenting', *Journal of Public Health Medicine*, 22(3), pp 337–42.

Kalra, N. and Newman, M. (2009) 'A systematic map of the research on the relationship between obesity and sedentary behaviour in young people. Technical report.' In: *Research Evidence in Education Library*, London: EPPI-Centre, Social Science Research Unit, Institute of Education, University of London.

Kavanagh, J., Stansfield, C. and Thomas, J. (2009) *Incentives to improve smoking, physical activity, dietary and weight management behaviours: a scoping review of the research evidence,* London: EPPI-Centre, Social Science Research Unit, Institute of Education, University of London.

Kelly, M.P., Speller, V. and Meyrick, J. (2004) *Getting evidence into practice in public health,* NICE, www.nice.org.uk/aboutnice/whoweare/aboutthehda/evidencebase/keypapers/evidenceintopractice/getting_evidence_into_practice_in_public_health.jsp.

Kempe, C.H., Silverman, F.N., Steele, B.F., Droegmueller, W. and Silver, H.K. (1962) 'The battered child syndrome', *Journal of the American Medical Association*, 181, pp 17–24.

Kempson, E. (1996) *Life on a low income,* York: York Publishing Services.

Kendrick, D., Coupland, C., Mulvaney, C.A., Simpson, J., Smith, S.J. and Sutton, A. (2007) 'Home safety education and provision of safety equipment for injury prevention', *Cochrane Database of Systematic Reviews 2007*, (1):CD005014.

Kennedy, I. (2010) *Getting it right for children and young people: overcoming cultural barriers in the NHS so as to meet their needs,* www.dh.gov.uk/prod_consum_dh/groups/dh_digitalassets/@dh/@en/@ps/documents/digitalasset/dh_119446.pdf.

Kirby, K. and Sopp, L. (1986) *Houses in multiple occupation in England and Wales: report of a postal survey of local authorities,* London: HMSO.

Kolvin, I., Miller, F.W. and Garside, R.F. (1983) 'A longitudinal study of deprivation: lifecycle changes in one generation – implications for the next generation', in M.H. Schmidt and H. Remschmidt (eds) *Epidemiology approaches in child psychiatry II*, Stuttgart and New York: G. Thieme.

Kuh, D., Hardy, R., Hotopf, M., Lawlor, D.A., Maughan, B., Westendorp, R.J., Cooper, R., Black, S. and Mishra, G. (2009) 'A review of lifetime risk factors for mortality', *British Actuarial Journal*, 15(Supplement), pp 17–64.

Kuper, S. (2009) 'The man who invented exercise', *Financial Times*, September 11.

Kurinczuk, J., Hollowell, J., Brocklehurst, P. and Gray, R. (2009) 'Infant mortality: overview and context', Inequalities in Infant Mortality Project, Briefing Paper no 1, Oxford: Perinatal Epidemiology Unit, University of Oxford.

Lancet (2011) '(Editorial) Urgently needed: a framework convention for obesity control', *Lancet*, 378(9739), p 741.

Lawlor, D.A. and Shaw, M. (2004) 'Teenage pregnancies – high compared with where and when ?' *Journal of the Royal Society of Medicine*, 97(3), pp 121–3.

Leach, P. (1997) *Getting positive about discipline: a guide for today's parents*, Barkingside: Barnardo's.

Lealman, G.T., Haigh, D., Phillips, J.M., Stone, J. and Ord-Smith, C. (1983) 'Prediction and prevention of child abuse – an empty hope?' *Lancet*, June 25, pp 1423–4.

Lester, S. and Maudsley, M. (2006) *Play, naturally: a review of children's natural play*. London: Children's Play Council. www.playday.org.uk/PDF/play-naturally-a-review-of-childrens-natural%20play.pdf.

Levin, H.M. (1978) 'A decade of policy developments in improving education and training for low-income populations', in T.R. Cook, M.L. Del Refario, K.M. Hinnegan, M.M. Mark and W.W.K. Trochim (eds) *Evaluation studies review annual*, 3, Beverley Hills: Sage.

Lister-Sharp, D., Chapman, S., Stewart-Brown, S. and Sowden, A. (1999) 'Health promoting schools and health promotion in schools: two systematic reviews', *Health Technology Assessment*, 3, pp 1–207.

Lloyd, E., Hemingway, M., Newman, T., Roberts H. and Webster, A. (1997) *Today and tomorrow: investing in children*, Barkingside: Barnardo's.

Lucas, P., Arai, L., Baird, J., Kleijnen, J., Law, C. and Roberts, H. (2007) 'A systematic review of lay views about infant size and growth', *Archives of Disease in Childhood*, 92, pp 120–7.

Lumley, J., Chamberlain, C., Dowswell, T., Oliver, S., Oakley, L. and Watson, L. (2009) 'Interventions for promoting smoking cessation during pregnancy', *Cochrane Database of Systematic Reviews 2009*, Issue 3, DOI: 10.1002/14651858. CD001055.pub3.

Lupton, C. and Nixon, P. (1999) *Empowering practice? A critical appraisal of the family group conference approach,* Bristol: The Policy Press

Lyons, R.A., John, A. and Brophy, S. (2006) 'Modification of the home environment for the reduction of injuries', *Cochrane Database of Systematic Reviews 2006*, (4):CD003600.

MacDonald, G. (2001a) 'Child protection', in T. Newman, D. McNeish and H. Roberts (eds) *What works in child care,* Oxford: Oxford University Press.

MacDonald, G (2001b) *Effective interventions for child abuse and neglect: an evidence-based approach to evaluating and planning interventions*, Chichester: John Wiley.

Macdonald, G. and Roberts, H. (1995) *What works in the early years? Effective interventions in health, social welfare, education and child protection*, Barkingside: Barnardo's.

Macdonald G. with Winkley, A. (2000) *What works in child protection?* Barkingside: Barnardo's.

Macdonald, G., Sheldon, B. and Gillespie, J. (1992) 'Contemporary studies of the effectiveness of social work', *British Journal of Social Work*, 22(6) pp 614–43.

Macfarlane, A.J. and Mugford, M. (2000) *Birth counts: statistics of pregnancy and childbirth: volume 1: text,* 2nd edition, London: The Stationery Office.

Macintyre, S. (2011) 'Good intentions and perceived wisdom are not good enough: the need for controlled trials in public health', *Journal of Epidemiology and Community Health,* 65, pp 564–7.

Mackenbach, J.P. (2011) 'Can we reduce health inequalities? An analysis of the English strategy (1997–2010) *Journal of Epidemiology and Community Health,* 65, pp 568–75.

MacMillan, H.L., Wathen, C.N., Barlow, J., Fergusson, D.M., Leventhal, J.M. and Taussig, H.N. (2009) 'Interventions to prevent child maltreatment and associated impairment', *Lancet,* 373 (9659) pp 250–66.

Marmot, M. (2010) *Fair society, healthy lives: strategic review of health inequalities in England post 2010,* London: Marmot review, www.instituteofhealthequity.org/Content/FileManager/pdf/fairsocietyhealthylives.pd, www.instituteofhealthequity.org/.

Marmot, G., Davey Smith, G., Stansfield, S., Patel, C., North, F., Head, J., White, I., Brunner, E. and Feeney, A. (1991) 'Health inequalities among British civil servants: the Whitehall II study', *Lancet,* 37 (8754), pp 1387–93.

Marmot, M., Allen, J. and Goldblatt, P. (2010) 'A social movement based on evidence, to reduce inequalities in health', *Social Science and Medicine,* vol 71, pp 1254-8.

Marsh, P. and Crow, G. (1998) *Family group conferences in child welfare,* Oxford: Blackwell Science.

Marteau, T.M., Ogilivie, D., Roland, M., Suhrcke, M. and Kelly, M.P. (2011) 'Judging nudging: can nudging improve population health?', *British Medical Journal,* 342: doi:10.1136/bmj.d228.

Mayall, B. (ed.) (1995) *Children's childhoods observed and experienced,* London: The Falmer Press.

McCord, J. (1981) 'Consideration of some effects of a counselling programme', in S.E. Martin, L.B. Sechrest and R. Redner (eds) *New directions in the rehabilitation of criminal offenders,* Washington, DC: National Academy Press.

McCormick, J. and Harrop, A. (2010) *Devolution's impact on low income people and places,* York: Joseph Rowntree Foundation.

McDonagh, M.S., Whiting, P.F., Wilson, P.M., Sutton, A.J., Chestnutt, I., Cooper, J., Misso, K., Bradley, M., Treasure, E. and Kleijnen, J. (2000) 'Systematic review of water fluoridation', *British Medical Journal,* 321, pp 855-9.

McMillan, M. (1904) *Education through the imagination,* London: Swan Sonnenschein and Co.

McNeish, D., Roberts, H. and Barrett, A. (1995) *The prevention of child accidents in Wardleworth, Rochdale,* Barkingside: Rochdale Borough Accident Prevention Group and Barnardo's.

Meadows, P. (2010) *National Evaluation of Sure Start local programmes: an economic perspective,* London: Department for Education.

Meltzer, H., Gatward, R., Corbin, T., Robert Goodman, R. and Ford, T. (2003) *The mental health of young people looked after by local authorities in England,* London: The Stationery Office, www.esds.ac.uk/doc/5280/mrdoc/pdf/5280userguide.pdf

Mermelstein, R. and the Tobacco Control Network Writing Group (1999) 'Explanations of ethnic and gender differences in youth smoking: a multisite qualitative investigation', *Nicotine and Tobacco Research,* 1, pp 591–8.

Middleton, S., Ashworth K. and Braithwaite I. (1997) *Small fortunes: spending on children, childhood poverty and parental sacrifice,* York: Joseph Rowntree Foundation.

Milne, R. and Law, C. (2009) 'The NIHR public health research programme: developing evidence for public health decision makers', *Journal of Public Health,* 31(4): 589–92.

Mishna, F., Cook, C., Saini, M., Wu, M.-J. and MacFadden, R. (2009) *Interventions for children, youth, and parents to prevent and reduce cyber abuse,* http://campbell collaboration.org/lib/download/681/.

Mitchell, J. (1984) *What is to be done about illness and health?,* Harmondsworth: Penguin.

Molloy, M. (2007) 'Volunteering as a community mother – a pathway to lifelong learning', *Community Practitioner,* 80(5), pp 26–32.

Mooney, A., Owen, C. and Statham, J. (2008) *Disabled children: numbers, characteristics and local service provision, Research Report 042,* London: DCSF.

More, R., Anderson, G.C. and Bergman, N. (2007) 'Early skin-to-skin contact for mothers and their healthy newborn infants', *Cochrane Database of Systematic Reviews 2007,* Issue 3, DOI: 10.1002/14651858.CD003519.pub2.

Morris, J. (1998) *Don't leave us out: involving disabled children and young people with communication impairments,* York: Joseph Rowntree Foundation.

MRC (2008) *Developing and evaluating complex interventions: new guidance,* London: Medical Research Council, www.mrc.ac.uk/complexinterventionsguidance.

Munro, E. (2011) *The Munro review of child protection: final report: a child-centred system,* www.education.gov.uk/munroreview/downloads/8875_DfE_Munro_ Report_TAGGED.pdf.

Munro, E. (2003) *Outcomes for looked after children: life pathways and decision making for very young children in care or accommodation,* Loughborough: Centre for Child and Family Research, www.lboro.ac.uk/research/ccfr/Publications/Evidence10.pdf.

Naidoo, J. (1984) *Evaluation of the Play it Safe Campaign in Bristol,* London: Child Accident Prevention Trust.

NCMP (2009/10) *National Child Measurement Programme,* www.esds.ac.uk/ findingData/snDescription.asp?sn=6789.

NESS team (2010) *The Impact of Sure Start local programmes on five year olds and their families,* London, Department for Education. www.ness.bbk.ac.uk/impact/ documents/RR067.f.

Newman, T. (2000) *Children and parental illness: a study in Merthyr Tydfil County Borough Council,* Barkingside: Barnardo's.

Newman, T. (2010) *Ensuring all disabled children and young people and their families receive services which are sufficiently differentiated to meet their diverse needs,* www.c4eo. org.uk/themes/disabledchildren/diverseneeds/files/c4eo_diverse_needs_kr_6. pdf.

Newman, T., McEwen, J., Mackin, H. and Slowley, M. (2010) *Improving the wellbeing of disabled children (up to age 8) and their families through increasing the quality and range of early years interventions,* Barkingside: Barnardo's Policy and Research Unit.

NHS CRD (1996) 'Preventing unintentional injuries in children and young adolescents', *Effective Health Care Bulletin,* 2(5), pp1–16.

NICE (2006a) *Report on NICE Citizens Council meeting: inequalities in health,* London: NICE, www.nice.org.uk/niceMedia/pdf/CitizensCouncilHealth InequalitiesReport0806.pdf.

NICE (2006b) *Obesity: the prevention, identification, assessment and management of overweight and obesity in adults and children,* London: NICE.

NICE (2008a) *Mass media and point of sales measures to prevent the uptake of smoking by children and young people,* London: NICE, Public Health Guidance.

NICE (2008b) *Intrapartum care: full guideline,* London: NICE. http://guidance. nice.org.uk/CG55/Guidance/pdf/Englh.

NICE (2008c) *Guidance on the promotion and creation of physical environments that support increased levels of physical activity: NICE public health guidance,* London: NICE. http://guidance.nice.org.uk/PH8.

NICE (2009) *When to suspect child maltreatment: full guideline,* http://guidance. nice.org.uk/CG89/Guidance/pdf/EngliCE.

NICE (2010) *Quitting smoking in pregnancy and following childbirth,* London: NICE, www.nice.org.uk/guidance/PH26.

NICE (2011) *Maternal and child nutrition,* http://guidance.nice.org.uk/PH11/ Guidance/doc/English.

NICE/SCIE (2010) *Promoting the quality of life of looked-after children and young people,* London: NICE.

Nutley, S.M. with Davies, H.T.O. and Walters, I. (2007) *Using evidence: how research can improve public services,* Bristol: The Policy Press.

Nye, C., Turner, H.M. and Schwartz, J. B. (2006) *Approaches to parental involvement for improving the academic performance of elementary school age children,* The Campbell Collaboration Library www.sfi.dk/graphics/Campbell/reviews/parental_ involvement_review.pdf.

Oakley, A. (1981) 'Interviewing women: a contradiction in terms?' in H. Roberts (ed.) *Doing feminist research,* London: Routledge and Kegan Paul.

Oakley, A. (1996) *Man and wife: Richard and Kay Titmuss: my parents' early years,* London: Harper Collins.

Oakley, A. (1998) 'A public policy experimentation: lessons from America', *Policy Studies,* 19(2), pp 93–114.

Oakley, A. (2000) *Experiments in knowing: gender and method in social sciences,* Cambridge: Polity Press.

O'Donnell, C.R. and Lydgate, T. (1979) 'The buddy system: review and follow-up', *Child Behavior Therapy,* 1, pp 161–9.

Olds, D., Henderson, C.R. Jr., Cole, R., Eckenrode, J., Kitzman, H., Luckey, D., Pettitt, L., Sidora, K., Morris, P. and Powers, J. (1998) 'Long-term effects of nurse home visitation on children's criminal and antisocial behavior: fifteen-year follow-up of a randomized controlled trial', *Journal of the American Medical Association,* 280, pp 1238–44.

Olds. L. , Henderson, C.R., Kitzman, H., Eckenrode, J., Cole, R. and Tatelbaum, R. (1999) 'Parental and infancy home visitation by nurses: recent findings', *The Future of Children,* http://futureofchildren.org/futureofchildren/publications/ docs/09_01_02.pdf.

Oliver, S., Thomas, J., Harden, A., Shepherd, J. and Oakley, A. (2006) 'Research synthesis for tackling health inequalities: lessons from methods developed within systematic reviews with a focus on marginalised groups', in A. Killoran, C. Swann and M. Kelly (eds) *Public health evidence: tackling health inequaliblic,* Oxford: Oxford University Press.

Orton, M. (2006) 'Wealth, citizenship and responsibility: the views of better off citizens in the UK', *Citizenship Studies,* 10 (2), pp 251–65.

Orton, M. and Rowlingson, K. (2007a) *Public attitudes towards income inequality,* York: Joseph Rowntree Foundation.

Orton, M. and Rowlingson, K. (2007b) 'A problem of riches: towards a new social policy research agenda on the distribution of economic resources', *Journal of Social Policy,* 36(1), pp 59–78.

Osborn, A.F. and Milbank, J.E. (1985) *The association of preschool educational experience with subsequent ability, attainment and behaviour: report to the Department of Education and Science,* Bristol: Department of Child Health, University of Bristol.

Oude, L.H., Baur, L., Jansen, H., Shrewsbury, V.A., O'Malley, C. and Stolk, R.P. (2009) 'Interventions for treating obesity in children', *Cochrane Database of Systematic Reviews 2009,* Issue 1. art no: CD001872. DOI:10.1002/14651858. CD001872.pub2.

Park, A., Curtice, J., Clery, E. and Bryson, C. (2011) *British social attitudes: the 27th report,* London: Sage.

Payne, H. and Butler, I. (1998) 'Improving the health care process and determining health outcomes for children looked after by the local authority', *Ambulatory Child Health,* 4, pp 165–72.

Petrosino, A., Turpin-Petrosino, C. and Buehler, J. (2002) '"Scared Straight" and other juvenile awareness programs for preventing juvenile deliquency', *Cochrane Database of Systematic Reviews,* Issue 2. art. no.: CD002796. DOI: 10.1002/14651858.CD002796.

Petticrew, M. (2001) 'Systematic reviews from astronomy to zoology: myths and misconceptions', *British Medical Journal,* 322, pp 98–101.

Petticrew, M. and Roberts, H. (2003) 'Evidence, hierarchies and typologies: horses for courses', *Journal of Epidemiology and Community Health,* 57, pp 527–9.

Petticrew, M. and Roberts, H. (2006) *Systematic reviews in the social sciences,* Oxford: Blackwell.

Phoenix, A. (1990) *Young mothers,* Cambridge: Polity.

Pilkington, B. and Kremer, J. (1995) 'A review of the epidemiological research on child sexual abuse: clinical samples', *Child Abuse Review,* 4, pp 191–205.

Pilkington, P. (2000) 'Reducing the speed limit to 20mph in urban areas', *British Medical Journal,* 32(7243), p 1160.

Platt, S.P., Martin, C.J. and Hunt, S.M. (1989) 'Damp housing, mould growth, and symptomatic health state', *British Medical Journal,* 201, pp 363–6.

Pless, B. (2002) 'Smoke detectors and house fires: alarms failed because detectors were not installed or maintained properly', *British Medical Journal,* 325, pp 979–80.

Plowden, S. and Hillman, M. (1996) *Speed control and transport policy,* London: Policy Studies Institute.

Polnay, L. (2000) 'Take it with a pillar of salt or "ambitious but achievable targets"', *Archives of Disease in Childhood*, 82(4), pp 278–9.

Polnay, L. and Ward, H. (2000) 'Promoting the health of looked after children', editorial, *British Medical Journal*, 320, pp 661–2.

Power, C. and Hertzman, C. (1997) 'Social and biological pathways linking early life and adult disease', *British Medical Bulletin*, 53, pp 210–21.

Power, C., Manor, O. and Fox, J. (1991) *Health and class: the early years*, London: Chapman and Hall.

Prescott-Clarke, P. and Primatesta, P. (eds) (1998) *Health survey for England: the health of young people '95–97*, London, The Stationery Office.

Quick, A. and Wilkinson, R. (1991) *Income and health*, London: Socialist Health Association.

Quigley, M.A., Kelly, Y.J. and Sacker, A. (2007) 'Infant feeding, solid foods and hospitalisation in the first 8 months after birth', *Archives of Diseases in Childhood*, 94, pp 148–50.

Rachman, S.J. and Wilson, G.T. (1980) *The effects of psychological therapy*, Oxford: Pergamon.

Rawlins, M. (2008) '*De testimonio*: on the evidence for decisions about the use of therapeutic interventions', *The Lancet*, 372(9656), pp 2152–61.

RCOG (2008) *Standards for maternity care*, London: Royal College of Obstetricians and Gynaecologists.

Read, J., Blackburn, C. and Spencer, N. (2010) 'Disabled children in the UK: a quality assessment of quantitative data sources', *Child: Care, Health and Development*, 36(1), pp 130–41.

Reading, R., Bissell, S. and Goldhagen, J, (2009) 'Promotion of children's rights and prevention of child maltreatment', *Lancet*, 373(9660), pp 332–43.

Rees, R., Kavanagh, J., Harden, A., Shepherd, J., Brunton, G., Oliver, S. and Oakley, A. (2006) 'Young people and physical activity: a systematic review matching their views to effective interventions', *Health Education Research*, 21(6), pp 806–25.

Rees, R., Oliver, K., Woodman, J. and Thomas, J. (2009) *Children's views about obesity, body size, shape and weight: a systematic review.* London: EPPI Centre, Social Science Research Unit, Institute of Education, University of London.

Reifsnider, E., Allan, J. and Percy, M. (2000) 'Mothers' explanatory models of lack of child growth', *Public Health Nursing*, 17, pp 434–42.

Reinisch, J.M. and Sanders, S. (1999) 'Would you say you "had sex" if…?' *Journal of the American Medical Association*, 281, pp 285–7.

Rice, C., Roberts H., Smith S.J. and Bryce C. (1994) 'It's like teaching your child to swim in a pool full of alligators: lay voices and professional research on child accidents', in J. Popay and G. Williams (eds) *Researching the people's health*, London: Routledge.

Richardson, J. and Joughin, C. (2000) *The mental health needs of looked after children*, London: Focus/Royal College of Psychiatrists/Gaskell.

Rickards, L., Fox, K., Roberts, C., Fletcher, L. and Goddard, E. (2004) *Living in Britain: results from the 2002 General Household survey*, London: The Stationery Office, www.ons.gov.uk/ons/dcp14763_170919.pdf.

Riley, T. and Hawe, P. (2009) 'A typology of practice narratives during the implementation of a preventive, community intervention trial', *Implementation Science*, 4:80, www.implementationscience.com/content/4/1/80.

Ritter, G., Denny, G., Albin, G., Barnett, J. and Blankenship, V. (2006) 'The effectiveness of volunteer tutoring programs: A systematic review' (PDF). *Campbell Systematic Reviews* 2006:7, www.givewell.org/files/unitedstates/campbell_academic%20achievement_tutoring.PDF.

Ritter, G., Barnett, J.H., Denny, G.S. and Albin, G.R. (2009) 'The effectiveness of volunteer tutoring programs for elementary and middle school students: a meta-analysis', *Review of Educational Research*, 79(1), pp 3–38.

Roberts, H. (2000) 'What is Sure Start?' *Archives of Disease in Childhood*, 82(6), pp 435–7.

Roberts, H. (2008a) 'Help, I'm ill', *Journal of Epidemiology and Community Health*, 62;572.

Roberts, H. (2008b) 'Disabled stretch limo', *Journal of Epidemiology and Community Health*, 62: 565 doi:10.1136/jech.2007.07193.

Roberts, H., Smith S.J. and Bryce C. (1993) 'Prevention is better ...', *Sociology of Health and Illness*, 15(4), pp 447–63.

Roberts, H., Smith, S. and Bryce, C. (1995) *Children at risk? Safety as a social value*, Buckingham: Open University Press.

Roberts, H., Curtis, K., Liabo, K., Rowland, D., DiGuiseppi, C. and Roberts, I. (2004a) 'Putting public health evidence into practice: increasing the prevalence of working smoke alarms in disadvantaged inner city housing', *Journal of Epidemiology and Community Health*, 58, pp 280–5.

Roberts, H., Liabo, K., Lucas, P., DuBois, D. and Sheldon, T.A. (2004b) 'Mentoring to reduce antisocial behaviour in childhood', *British Medical Journal*, 328(7438), pp 512–4.

Roberts, H., Shiell, A. and Stevens, M. (2008) 'What works, what counts and what matters? Communities of practice as a locus for contributing to resource allocation decisions' in Le May (ed.) *Communities of practice in health and social care*, Oxford: Blackwell.

Roberts, H. Smith, S.J., Campbell, B. and Rice, C. (2010) 'Safety as a social value: re-visiting a participatory case study in Scotland', in M. Kirst, N. Schaefer-McDaniel and S. Hwang (eds) *Converging disciplines: a transdisciplinary approach to urban health problems*, New York: Springer.

Roberts, I. and Coggan, C. (1994) 'Blaming children for child pedestrian injuries', *Social Science and Medicine*, 38(5), pp 749–53.

Roberts, I. and Power, C. (1996) 'Does the decline in child injury mortality vary by social class? A comparison of class specific mortality in 1981 and 1991', *British Medical Journal*, 313, pp 784–6.

Roberts, I., Ashton T., Dunn R. and Lee-Joe, T. (1994) 'Preventing child pedestrian injury: pedestrian education or traffic calming?' *Australian Journal of Public Health*, 18(2), pp 209–12.

Roberts I., Kramer M.S. and Suissa S. (1996) 'Does home visiting prevent childhood injury? A systematic review of randomised controlled trials', *British Medical Journal*, 312, pp 29–33.

Rose, G. and Day, S. (1990) 'The population mean predicts the number of deviant individuals', *British Medical Journal*, 310, pp 1031–4.

Rosenberg, W. and Donald, A. (1995) 'Evidence based medicine: an approach to clinical problem-solving', *British Medical Journal*, 310, pp 1122–6.

Rothon, C., Head, J., Klineberg, E. and Stansfeld, S. (2011) 'Can social support protect bullied adolescents from adverse outcomes? A prospective study on the effects of bullying on the educational achievement and mental health of adolescents at secondary schools in East London', *Journal of Adolescence,* 34(3), pp 579–88.

Rowland, D., DiGuiseppi, C., Roberts, I., Curtis, K., Roberts, H., Ginnelly, L., Sculpher, M. and Wade, A. (2002) 'Prevalence of working smoke alarms in local authority inner city housing: randomised controlled trial', *British Medical Journal*, 325, pp 998–1001.

Rowlingson, K., Orton, M. and Taylor, E. (2010) 'Do we still care about inequality?' in A. Park, J. Curtice, E. Clery and C. Bryson (eds) *British social attitudes: the 27th report: exploring Labour's legacy,* London: Sage Publications, pp 1–28.

Rush, B., Sheill, A. and Hawe, P. (2004) 'A census of economic evaluations of health promotion', *Health Education Research*, 19(6):707-719.

Rychetnik, L., Frommer, M., Hawe, P. and Shiell, A. (2002) 'Criteria for evaluating evidence on public health interventions', *Journal of Epidemiology and Community Health,* 56, pp 119-127.

Salariya, E.N., Easton, P.M. and Cater, J.I. (1978) 'Duration of breastfeeding after early initiation and frequent feeding', *Lancet*, 2, pp 1141–3.

Schweinhart, L. and Weikart, D. (1993) *A summary of significant benefits: the High-Scope Perry Pre-school Study through age 27,* Ypsilanti, MI and UK: High/Scope.

Schweinhart, L. and Weikart, D. (1997) *Lasting differences: the High/Scope preschool curriculum comparison study through age 23,* High/Scope Educational Research Foundation Monograph No. 12. Ypsilanti, MI: High/Scope Press.

Scott, S. (1998) 'Fortnightly review: aggressive behaviour in childhood', *British Medical Journal*, 316, pp 202–6.

Scott, S. Knapp, M., Henderson, J. and Maughan, B. (2001) 'Financial cost of social exclusion: follow up study of antisocial children into adulthood', *British Medical Journal,* 323, p 191.

Sefton, T. (2005) 'Give and take: public attitudes to redistribution', in A. Park, J. Curtice, K. Thomson, C. Bromley, M. Phillips and M. Johnson (eds) *British Social Attitudes: 22nd report*, London: Sage.

Shaw, M., Dorling, D., Gordon D. and Davey Smith, G. (1999) *The widening gap: health inequalities and policy in Britain*, Bristol: The Policy Press.

Sheldon, T.A., Guyatt, G.H. and Haines, A. (1998) 'Getting research findings into practice: when to act on the evidence', *British Medical Journal*, 317, pp 139–42.

Shemilt, I., Mugford, M,. Moffatt, P., Harvey, I., Reading, R., Shepstone, L. and Belderson, P. (2004) 'A national evaluation of school breakfast clubs: where does economics fit in?' *Child: Care, Health and Development,* 30(5), pp 429–37.

Shemilt, I., Mugford, M., Vale, L., Marsh, K. and Donaldson, C. (eds) (2010) *Evidence-based decisions and economics: health care, social welfare, education and criminal justice,* Oxford: BMJ Books/Wiley-Blackwell.

Shiell, A., Hawe, P. and Gold, L. (2008) 'Complex interventions or complex systems? Implications for health economic evaluation', *British Medical Journal,* 336, pp 1281–3.

SIGN (2010) *Management of obesity: quick reference guide,* Edinburgh: Scottish Intercollegiate Guidelines Network, www.sign.ac.uk/pdf/qrg115.pdf.

Silverman, W.A. (1980) *Retrolental fibroplasia: a modern parable,* New York: Grune and Stratton.

Skrabanek, P. (1990) 'Why is preventive medicine exempted from ethical constraints?' *Journal of Medical Ethics,*16, pp 187–90.

Skuse, T. and Ward, H. (1999) 'Current research findings about the health of looked after children', paper presented to: *Quality Protects Seminar: Improving Health Outcomes for Looked After Childre*n, 6 December, Dartington: Social Research Unit and Loughborough University.

Sloper, P. (1999) 'Models of service support for parents of disabled children: what do we know? What do we need to know?' *Child: Care Health and Development,* 25(2), pp 85–99, www.aafesp.org.br/biblioteca/AtencaoSaude/models_of_service_support.pdf .

Smith, L., Draper, E,. Manktelow, B. and Field, D. (2009) 'Socio-economic differences in survival and provision of neonatal care: population-based study of very pre-term infants', *British Medical Journal,* 339:b4702.

Smith, N. (2010) 'Islington Career Start: how Islington's employment scheme has improved the transitions to adulthood for looked after young people and care leavers', *Outcome Network,* 2, www.outcome-network.org/journal_issues.

Smith, P., Talamelli, L., Cowie, H., Naylor, P. and Chauhan, P. (2004) 'Profiles of non-victims, escaped victims, continuing victims and new victims of school bullying', *British Journal of Educational Psychology,* 74, pp 565–81.

Smith, R. (1996) 'Keeping the bad news from journalists', *British Medical Journal,* 314, p 8.

Smith, R. (2002) (letter) 'Why studies on smoke alarms are important and why "feckless" is a loaded word', *British Medical Journal,* www.bmj.com/content/325/7371/979.full/reply#bmj_el_26666.

Spencer, N. (2000) *Poverty and child health,* Abingdon: Radcliffe Memorial Press.

Spencer, N. (2006) 'Social equalization in youth: evidence from a cross-sectional British survey', *European Journal of Public Health,*16, pp 368–75.

Spencer, N., Blackburn, C.M. and Read, J.M.((2010) 'Prevalence and social patterning of limiting long-term illness/disability in children and young people under the age of 20 years in 2001: UK census-based cross-sectional study', *Child: Care, Health and Development,* 36(4), pp 566–73.

St James-Roberts, I. and Samlal Singh, C. (2001) *Can mentors help primary school children with behaviour problems? Final report of the Thomas Coram Research Unit between March 1997 and 2000,* London: Home Office.

Stein, M. (2010) *Vulnerable children knowledge review 3: increasing the number of care leavers in settled, safe accommodation,* London: C4EO.

Steinbach, R., Grundy, C., Edwards, P., Wilkinson, P. and Green, J. (2010) 'The impact of 20 mph traffic speed zones on inequalities in road casualties in London', *Journal of Epidemiology and Community Health,* doi:10.1136/jech.2010.112193.

Stevens, M., Roberts, H. and Shiell, A. (2010) 'Research review: economic evidence for interventions in children's social care: revisiting the What Works for Children project', *Child and Family Social Work,* 15, pp 145–54.

Stewart-Brown, S. (2006) *What is the evidence on school health promotion in improving health or preventing disease and, specifically, what is the effectiveness of the health promoting schools approach?* Copenhagen: WHO Regional Office for Europe, www.euro. who.int/document/e88185.pdf.

Stone, D. (1993) *Costs and benefits of accident prevention: a selective review of the literature,* Glasgow: Public Health Research Unit, University of Glasgow.

Sundell, K. and Vinnerljung, B. (2004) 'Outcome of family group conferencing in Sweden: a 3 year follow-up', *Child Abuse and Neglect,* 28(3), pp 267–87.

Sutherland, H., Hancock, R., Hills, J. and Zantomio, F. (2008) *Keeping up or falling behind? The impact of benefit and tax uprating on incomes and poverty,* ISER Working Paper, 2008-18, Colchester: ISER.

Sutton, L., Smith, N., Deardon, C. and Middelton, S. (2007) *A child's eye view of social difference,* York: Joseph Rowntree Foundation.

Sweeney, L. and Haney, C. (1992) 'The influence of race on sentencing: a meta-analytic review of experimental studies', *Behavioral Sciences and the Law,* 10, pp 179–95.

Sweeting, H. and West, P. (1995) 'Family life and health in adolescence: a role for culture in the health inequalities debate?' *Social Science and Medicine,* 40, pp 163–75.

SWIA (2006) *Extraordinary lives,* Edinburgh: Social Work Inspection Agency.

Swinburn, B.A., Sacks, G., Hall, K.D., McPherson, K., Finegood, D.T., Moodie, M.L., and Gortmaker, S.L. (2011) 'The global obesity pandemic: shaped by global drivers and local environments', *Lancet,* 378, pp 804–14.

Tanne, J.H. (1999) 'JAMA's editor fired over sex article', *British Medical Journal,* www.bmj.com/content/318/7178/213.1.full.

Tarling, R., Burrows, J. and Clarke, A. (2001) *Dalston youth project part II (11-14): an evaluation,* London: Home Office.

Teare, L., Cookson, B. and Stone, S. (2001) 'Hand hygiene', *British Medical Journal,* 323, pp 411–12.

Thaler, R.H. and Sunstein, C.R. (2008) *Nudge: improving decisions about health, wealth, and happiness,* New Haven, CT: Yale University Press.

Thomas, B. and Dorling, D. (2004) *Know your place: housing wealth and inequality in Great Britain 1980–2003 and beyond,* London: Shelter.

Thompson, M. and Westreich, R. (1989) 'Restriction of mother infant contact in the immediate postnatal period', in I. Chalmers, M. Enkin and M.J.C. Keirse (eds) *Effective care in pregnancy and childbirth*, Oxford: Oxford University Press, pp 1322–30.

Thomson, H., Atkinson, R., Petticrew, M. and Kearns, A. (2006) 'Do urban regeneration programmes improve public health and reduce health inequalities? A synthesis of the evidence from UK policy and practice (1980–2004)' *Journal of Epidemiology and Community Health*, 60, pp 108-15.

Thurlbeck, S. (2000) 'Growing up in Britain' (review), *British Medical Journal*, 320, p 809.

Tickell, C. (2011) *The early years: foundations for life, health and learning: an independent report on the early years foundation stage to Her Majesty's Government*, http://media.education.gov.uk/MediaFiles/B/1/5/%7BB15EFF0D-A4DF-4294-93A1-1E1B88C13F68%7DTickell%20review.pdf.

Titmuss, R. (1943) *Birth, poverty and wealth*, London: Hamish Hamilton.

TNS Social (2009) *Sure Start Children's Centres: survey of parents*, London: DCSF, www.education.gov.uk/publications/eOrderingDownload/DCSF-RR083.pdf.

Towner, E., Dowswell, T. and Jarvis S. (1993) *The effectiveness of health promotion interventions in the prevention of unintentional childhood injury: a review of the literature*, London: Health Education Authority.

Towner, E., Dowswell, T., Mackereth, C. and Jarvis, S. (2001) *What works in preventing unintentional injuries in children and young adolescents?* London: Health Development Agency.

Tudor Hart, J. (1971) 'The inverse care law', *Lancet*, 297, pp 405–412.

Tudor Hart, J. (1988) *A new kind of doctor*, London: Merlin Press, p.10.

Turner, C., Spinks, A., McClure, R. and Nixon, J. (2004) 'Community-based interventions for the prevention of burns and scalds in children', *Cochrane Database of Systematic Reviews 2004*, (2):CD00433.

UNICEF (2000) *A league table of child poverty in rich nations*, Innocenti Report Card No 1, UNICEF, Innocenti Research Centre, Florence, Italy.

UNICEF (2003) *The state of the world's children 2002*. New York: UNICEF.

UNICEF (2004) *The State of the world's children: girls, education and development, 2003*. New York: UNICEF,

UNICEF (2005) *The state of the world's children: childhood under threat, 2004*. New York: UNICEF.

UNICEF (2006) *The state of the world's children: excluded and invisible, 2005*. New York: UNICEF.

University of Wisconsin (2002–5) *Program development and evaluation*, www.uwex.edu/ces/pdande/evaluation/evallogicmodel.html.

Utting, D. and Vennard, J. (2000) *What works with youth offenders in the community?* Barkingside: Barnardo's.

Vignoles, A. and Machin, S. (eds) *What's the good of education? The economics of education in the UK*, Princeton and Oxford: Princeton University Press.

Viner, R.M. and Barker, M. (2005) 'Young people's health: the need for action', *British Medical Journal*, 330 : 901, doi: 10.1136/bmj.330.7496.901.

Viner, R.M. and Taylor, B. (2005) 'Adult health and social outcomes of children who have been in public care: population-based study', *Pediatrics*, 115(4) 894–9.

Viner, R.M., Coffey, C., Mathers, C., Bloem, P., Costello, A., Santelli, J. and Patton, G.C. (2011) '50-year mortality trends in children and young people: a study of 50 low-income, middle-income, and high-income countries', *Lancet*, 377(9772), pp 1162–74.

Viudes, A. (2002) *Economic evaluation of the provision of area wide traffic calming schemes designed to prevent accidents in urban areas in the whole of England and Wales,* London: School of Hygiene and Tropical Medicine.

Wade, J., Biehal, N., Farrelly, N. and Sinclair, I. (2010) *Maltreated children in the looked after system: a comparison of outcomes for those who go home and those who do not,* London: Department for Education.

Wadsworth, M.E.J. (1991) *The imprint of time: childhood, history and adult life,* Oxford: Oxford University Press.

Wakefield, M., Chaloupka, F., Kaufman N.J., Orleans, C.T., Barker, D. and Ruel, E. (2000) 'Effect of restrictions on smoking at home, at school, and in public places on teenage smoking: cross sectional study', *British Medical Journal*, 321, pp 333–7.

Ward, H., Brown, R. and Westlake, D. (2012) *Safeguarding babies and very young children from abuse and neglect,* London: JKP.

Waters, E., Priest N., Armstrong, R., Oliver, S., Baker, P., McQueen, D., Summerbell, C., Kelly, M.P. and Swinburn, B. (2007) 'The role of a prospective public health intervention study register in building public health evidence: proposal for content and use', *Journal of Public Health Medicine*, 29(3), pp 322–7.

Watt, R.G. (2007) 'From victim blaming to upstream action: tackling the social determinants of oral health inequalities', *Community Dentistry and Oral Epidemiology*, 35(1), pp 1–11.

Webster, D. and Mackie, A. (1996) *A review of traffic calming schemes in 20mph zones,* TRRL report 215, Crowthorne: Transport and Road Research Laboratory.

Webster-Stratton, C. (1990) 'Long-term follow-up of families with young conduct problem children: from preschool to grade school', *Journal of Clinical Child Psychology*, 19, pp 144–9.

Wellings, K. and Kane, R. (1999) 'Trends in teenage pregnancy in England and Wales: how can we explain them?' *Journal of the Royal Society of Medicine*, 92, pp 277–82.

West, P. (1997) 'Health inequalities in the early years: is there equalisation in youth?' *Social Science and Medicine*, 44, pp 833–58.

Whitehead, M. and Popay, J. (2010) 'Swimming upstream? Taking action on the social determinants of health inequalities', *Social Science and Medicine,* 71, pp 1234–6.

Whitlock, E.P., O'Connor, E.A., Williams, S.B., Beil, T.L. and Lutz, K.W. (2010) 'Effectiveness of weight management interventions in children: a targeted systematic review for the USPSTF', *Pediatrics*, 125:e396–e418.

WHO (2008) *Inequities are killing people on grand scale, reports WHO's Commission,* www.who.int/mediacentre/news/releases/2008/pr29/en/index.html.

Widdowson, E.M. (1951) 'Mental contentment and physical growth', *The Lancet*, June 16, pp 316–18.

Wiggins, M., Bonell, C., Sawtell, M., Austerberry, H., Burchett, H., Allen, E. and Strange, V. (2009) 'Health outcomes of youth development programme in England: prospective matched comparison study', *British Medical Journal*, July 7, 339:b2534.

Wilkinson, R.G. (1994) *Unfair shares: the effects of widening income differences on the welfare of the young*, Barkingside: Barnardo's.

Wilkinson, R.G. and Pickett, K. (2009) *The spirit level: why more equal societies almost always do better*, London: Penguin.

Williams, H. and Sibert, J. (1983) 'Medicine and the media', *British Medical Journal*, 286, p 1893.

Wilson, P.M. and Sheldon, T.A. (2006) 'Muddy waters: evidence-based policy making, uncertainty and the "York review" on water fluoridation', *Evidence and Policy*, 2(3), pp 321–31.

Woodman, J., Lorenc, T., Harden, A. and Oakley, A. (2008) *Social and environmental interventions to reduce childhood obesity: a systematic map of reviews*, London: EPPI-Centre, Social Science Research Unit, Institute of Education, University of London.

Working Group on Inequalities in Health (1980) *Inequalities in health: report of a research working group*, (Black report), London: DHSS.

World Bank (2011) Mortality rate (infant) per 1000 live births, http://data.worldbank.org/indicator/SP.DYN.IMRT.IN.

Wright, C.M., Parker, L., Lamont, D. and Craft, A.W. (2001) 'Implications of childhood obesity for adult health: findings from thousand families cohort study', *British Medical Journal*, 323(7324), pp 1280–4.

Zelizer, V. (1994) *Pricing the priceless child: the changing social value of children*. Princeton, NJ: Princeton University Press.

Zoritch, B., Roberts I. and Oakley, A. (2000) 'Day care for pre-school children' *Cochrane Database of Systematic Reviews*, Issue 3, DOI: 10.1002/14651858. CD000564.

Web and other resources

Child health data and Healthy Child Programme

Child and Maternal Health Observatory

The national Child and Maternal Health Observatory (ChiMat) provides information and intelligence to improve decision making for high-quality, cost-effective services. It supports policy makers, commissioners, managers, regulators, and other health stakeholders working on children's, young people's and maternal health.
➤ www.chimat.org.uk

Healthy Child Programme: pregnancy and the first five years of life

The Healthy Child Programme for the early life stages focuses on a universal preventative service, providing families with a programme of screening, immunisation, health and development reviews, supplemented by advice around health, well-being and parenting.
➤ www.dh.gov.uk/en/Publicationsandstatistics/Publications/Publications PolicyAndGuidance/DH_107563

Healthy Child Programme from 5 to 19 years old

The Healthy Child Programme from 5 to 19 years old sets out the recommended framework of universal and progressive services for children and young people to promote optimal health and well-being. It outlines suggested roles and responsibilities for commissioners, health, education, local authority and other partners to encourage the development of high-quality services. As the operating framework for the NHS in England 2010/11 sets out, primary care trusts will want to review their service offer in line with *Healthy lives, brighter futures* (Department of Health, 2009). The Programme sets out support for giving children and their families the best start in life.
➤ www.dh.gov.uk/en/Publicationsandstatistics/Publications/Publications PolicyAndGuidance/DH_107566

Policy across the UK

4 Nations Child Policy Network was established in 2001 following devolution to provide accessible information on child policy developments from across the UK. The Network is a partnership between Children in Scotland, Children in Northern Ireland, Children in Wales and the National Children's Bureau. It provides access to information on child policy developments from each of the four nations of the United Kingdom.
> http://childpolicyinfo.childreninscotland.org.uk/
> www.ci–ni.org.uk/
> www.childreninwales.org.uk/
> www.ncb.org.uk/

Policy reports

Among the important policy reports related to inequalities in child health are:

Black report (1980) *Inequalities in health: report of a research working group* The Working Group on Inequalities in Health, was set up in 1977 to review information about differences in health status between the social classes; to consider possible causes and the implications for policy; and to suggest further research. The full text of the report appears on this website, along with interpretive material relating to a report set up by one government but received by the next.
> www.sochealth.co.uk/Black/black.htm

Acheson report (1998) *Independent enquiry into inequalities in health report* The Independent Enquiry into Inequalities in Health, was commissioned by the then government to contribute to the development of strategy for health and action on inequalities.
> www.dh.gov.uk/en/Publicationsandstatistics/Publications/Publications PolicyAndGuidance/DH_4097582

Commission on Social Determinants of Health (2008) *Closing the gap in a generation: health equity through action on the social determinants of health*, was established by the World Health Organization as a response to increasing concern about these persisting and widening inequities. Its three overarching recommendations were to improve daily living conditions; to tackle the inequitable distribution of power, money and resources; and to measure and understand the problem and assess the impact of action. A series of articles in *Social Science and Medicine* (2010, volume 71) respond to and comment on the report.
> www.who.int/social_determinants/thecommission/en/

Marmot review (2010) *Fair society, healthy lives: strategic review of health inequalities in England post 2010*, was an independent review into health inequalities in England.
> www.instituteofhealthequity.org/

Field report (2010) *The foundation years: preventing poor children becoming poor adults: the report of the Independent Review on Poverty and Life Chances* is an independent review on poverty and life chances, and makes recommendations on 'potential action by government and other institutions to reduce poverty and enhance life chances for the least advantaged, consistent with the Government's fiscal strategy'.
➤ http://webarchive.nationalarchives.gov.uk/20110120090128/
➤ http://povertyreview.independent.gov.uk/media/20254/poverty-report.pdf

Allen report (2011) *Early intervention: the next steps: an independent report to Her Majesty's Government* recommended early intervention as 'an approach which offers our country a real opportunity to make lasting improvements in the lives of our children, to forestall many persistent social problems and end their transmission from one generation to the next, and to make long-term savings in public spending'.
➤ www.dwp.gov.uk/docs/early-intervention-next-steps.pdf

Kennedy report (2010) *Getting it right for children and young people: overcoming cultural barriers in the NHS so as to meet their needs* was 'carried out amid widespread concern about the services provided by the NHS to children and young people' and concluded that 'Children and young people receive a disproportionately lower priority than adults in the imperatives of management and delivery, in the relative funding allocated, and in the realisation that investment in the care of children and young people will reduce the cost of care later in life'; 'We must invest to save and we must invest because it is right to do so.'
➤ www.dh.gov.uk/prod_consum_dh/groups/dh_digitalassets/@dh/@en/@ps/documents/digitalasset/dh_119446.pdf

Munro report (2011) *The Munro review of child protection: final report: a child-centred system* made recommendations 'to reform the child protection system from being over-bureaucratised and concerned with compliance to one that keeps a focus on children, checking whether they are being effectively helped, and adapting when problems are identified'.
➤ www.education.gov.uk/munroreview/downloads/8875_DfE_Munro_Report_TAGGED.pdf

Tickell report (2011) *The early years: foundations for life, health and learning: an independent report on the early years foundation stage to Her Majesty's Government* recommended that 'a greater emphasis is given in the EYFS to the role of parents and carers as partners in their children's learning'.
➤ http://media.education.gov.uk/MediaFiles/B/1/5/%7BB15EFF0D-A4DF-4294-93A1-1E1B88C13F68%7DTickell%20review.pdf

Where to go for good evidence

NHS Evidence

This is a service managed by the National Institute for Health and Clinical Excellence (NICE) that enables access to authoritative evidence and best practice. It is designed to help people from across the NHS, public health and social care sectors to make better decisions.
➤ www.evidence.nhs.uk/

Getting public health evidence into practice

A key reference on this topic remains Kelly et al. (2004), which addresses:

• What is the best way to develop evidence in public health?
• What is the definition of evidence?
• How may evidence best be used to produce guidance for practice?
• What are the practicalities involved in putting evidence into practice?
• What are the best ways of stimulating change in practice?
➤ www.nice.org.uk/aboutnice/whoweare/aboutthehda/evidencebase/keypapers/evidenceintopractice/getting_evidence_into_practice_in_public_health.jsp

The Cochrane Collaboration

The Cochrane Collaboration is an international organisation concerned with the preparation and maintenance of systematic reviews of health care interventions, and with making these accessible to end users, including clinicians, patients and researchers. The main work of the Collaboration is done by collaborative review groups, which have responsibility for supporting the preparation and maintenance of reviews in specific areas (usually health problems). Cochrane collaborative review groups provide:

• co-ordination of potential reviewers, who are often geographically scattered;
• methodological support to help reviewers minimise bias in reviews;
• practical support to reviewers through the development of specialised registers using sensitive electronic and hand searching for relevant studies;
• a framework for peer reviewing, editing, publishing and updating protocols and systematic reviews.
➤ www.cochrane.org

The following Cochrane groups are particularly relevant to thinking about inequalities in child health.

Cochrane Child Health Field has a vision that decision makers (health care providers, policymakers, parents and children/youth) concerned with child health make evidence-informed health care decisions by using high-quality Cochrane systematic reviews of the best available evidence.
➤ www.cochranechildhealth.ualberta.ca/

Cochrane Public Health Review Group is particularly interested in population-level interventions and reviews which tackle the determinants of health, including education, transport and food access and supply.
➤ http://ph.cochrane.org/

Cochrane Developmental, Psychosocial and Learning Problems Group, includes reviews of parenting programmes.
➤ http://dplpg.cochrane.org/

Cochrane Injuries Group tackles an area where there are huge inequalities in health.
➤ http://injuries.cochrane.org/

Cochrane Effective Practice and Organisation Care Group focuses on reviews of interventions designed to improve professional practice and the delivery of effective health services. This includes various forms of continuing education, quality assurance, informatics, and financial, organisational and regulatory interventions that can affect the ability of health care professionals to deliver services more effectively and efficiently.
➤ http://epoc.cochrane.org/

Cochrane/Campbell Equity Group encourages authors of both Campbell and Cochrane reviews to include explicit descriptions of the effects of the interventions not only on the whole population but on disadvantaged people, and/or to describe their ability to reduce socioeconomic inequalities in health and to promote their use to the wider community. Ultimately, this will help build the evidence base on such interventions and increase our capacity to act on the health gap between rich and poor.
➤ http://equity.cochrane.org/

Campbell Collaboration helps people make well-informed decisions by preparing, maintaining and disseminating systematic reviews in education, crime and justice, and social welfare.
➤ www.campbellcollaboration.org/

C4EO

The Centre for Excellence and Outcomes in Children and Young People's Services (C4EO) provides a range of products and support services to improve outcomes. It draws on a consortium of core partners: National Children's Bureau, National Foundation for Educational Research, Research in Practice and the Social Care Institute for Excellence.
➤ www.c4eo.org.uk/default.aspx

The EPPI Centre

The EPPI-Centre conducts systematic reviews of research evidence across a range of different topic areas and provides support for others who are undertaking systematic reviews or using research evidence.

They have a large number of systematic reviews in the fields of education, health promotion and public health. The Knowledge Pages on their website enable access to the key messages about a specific subject area, e.g. obesity, and may come from multiple reviews. The Reviews Search page provides a facility for searching the body of reviews available to date or browsing the full list of titles currently available
➤ http://eppi.ioe.ac.uk/cms/Default.aspx?tabid=56

National Children's Bureau Highlights

A well-respected series of summaries of important issues in social work and social care practice with children. Recent titles include:
The impact of domestic violence on children (2010)
Young people, online gaming and addiction (2010)
School leadership for well-being (2010)
➤ www.ncb.org.uk/cpis/resources/highlights

SCIE

Social Care Institute for Excellence (SCIE) is an independent charity working with adults, families and children's social care and social work services across the UK. They work closely with related services such as health care and housing. They gather and analyse knowledge about what works and translate that knowledge into practical resources, learning materials and services.
➤ www.scie.org.uk/

Poverty and inequality

The **Department for Work and Pensions** and the **Department for Education** deal with child poverty in the UK.
➤ www.dwp.gov.uk/policy/child-poverty/
➤ www.education.gov.uk/childrenandyoungpeople/families/childpoverty/a0066302/the-child-poverty-act

Poverty Site provides statistics and reports on poverty and social exclusion in the UK.
➤ www.poverty.org.uk/

Child Poverty Action Group campaigns for the abolition of poverty in the UK and a better deal for low income families with children.
➤ www.cpag.org.uk/

Equality Trust is an independent, evidence-based campaigning organisation working to reduce income inequality in order to improve the quality of life in the UK.
➤ www.equalitytrust.org.uk/about/aims

Resources for young people

Among the resources for young people touching on the subjects of this book are the following:

Who Cares Trust is a voice for children in care. It has a child-friendly website for children in the care system, explaining everything from the meaning of unfamiliar terms to what they can expect, and case studies of work placements.
➤ www.thewhocarestrust.org.uk/who-cares-town/index-council.php

Making Ourselves Heard is a national project to ensure that disabled children's right to be heard becomes a reality. It gives disabled children direct access to government and policy makers and ensures that the voices of disabled children and their success stories are heard. As well as involving children, it:

* supports professionals to encourage disabled children's participation;
* publicises good examples of where disabled children are involved in decision making;
* raises awareness of disability equality by promoting positive images of disability in childhood;
* promotes the inclusion of disabled children and young people in organisations that work with all children and young people.

➤ http://councilfordisabledchildren.org.uk/what-we-do/networks-campaigning/making-ourselves-heard

Royal College of Paediatrics and Child Health is committed to the safe, meaningful and ethical participation of children and young people and has a website to support this.
➤ www.rcpch.ac.uk/participation

What does it all mean?

A glossary of useful terms used in studies and systematic reviews can be accessed at
➤ www.cochrane.org/glossary/5

Index

The letter 'f' following a page number indicates a figure and 't' a table